AUDREY

THE TRUE STORY OF ONE CHILD'S HEROIC JOURNEY OF FAITH

BY GLORIA CONDE

year of
FAITH 2013 ~ Ave Maria

May Audrey's joyful spirit
be with you. May Christ
Jesus' powerful touch heal
you. May Mary's comfort
embrace you. And May
the Holy Angels protect
and lead you in the
way of salvation !!!
Peace in Jesus & Mary!

Cover and interior design by Joseph Hilliman | www.jhilliman.com

Translated from the French edition and edited by Trish Bailey

Library of Congress Cataloging-in-Publication Data
Conde, Gloria, 1966-
[Audrey. English]
Audrey : the true story of one child's heroic journey of faith / by Gloria Conde ; [translated from the French edition and edited by Trish Bailey]. — 1st ed.
p. cm.
ISBN 978-1-933271-18-7
1. Stevenson, Audrey, 1983-1991. 2. Catholic children—Religious life. 3. Leukemia in children—Patients—Religious life. 4. Catholic children—Biography. 5. Leukemia in children—Patients—Biography. I. Bailey, Trish. II. Title.

BX4705.S75C6613 2008
282'.46092—dc22
[B]

2008026647

PRINTED IN THE UNITED STATES OF AMERICA

8 7 6 5 4 3 2

Thanks to all those who have contributed to making this book a reality. Thank you, Lillian. Thank you, Jerome. Thank you to those young faces I know so well who have been asking for months: "When will the book about Audrey come out?"

TABLE OF CONTENTS

TABLE Of CONTENTS

TABLE OF CONTENTS

FOREWORD

"My Little Carmelite" is how I like to refer to Audrey.

It helps me when I need reminding that God has no regard for age when dispensing his gifts, and true wisdom is not a fruit of years lived, nor is it the product of reason alone. And especially I like to call her by this name when asking her help for favors, above all when these have to do with vocations.

You don't have to have met Audrey for her to become part of your life. The closest I ever came to meeting her was through a photograph of her in her PJs in a hospital bed and my conversations with Jerome, her dad. It was Jerome who gave me the photograph, and between puffs of the ever-present (at the time) cigarette, told me about his daughter being in hospital. It was that curious and uplifting mixture of a parent's deep pain, pride, hope, love, and resignation that many priests have occasion to perceive in the heart and words of believing folk touched by tragedy—the times we think God has suddenly changed all the parameters only to discover that he hasn't changed anything at all; he has done no more than remind us of the true parameters.

We love children, and we enjoy them because, more than anywhere else, in them we see the future. And since they are still lively, innocent, and spontaneous, vessels of God's grace, we are made to think that the future will be much better and much brighter. And then suddenly God simply acts like God without asking our permission, and we discover that in the presence of the Ever-Present, the present is all that matters.

When you read the pages that follow you will see how Audrey was privileged to have that heightened sense of God's presence, and how that led her to do things "here and now" (learning her French verb tables, doing a sacrifice to console Jesus...).

Simple things mostly—some extraordinary upon reflection—but how many of us dared to do them when we were little, and how many of us do them well now? But the most winning thing about Audrey is that she doesn't lecture you. She just seems to invite you to sit down on that hospital bed beside her, she cuddles up to you like any little girl her age, and with the simplicity and depth of her actions she invites you and shows you how to love more sincerely, more simply, more completely.

I hope this book will be like that for you. Rather than a biography, it is a series of vignettes in chronological order that I am sure will win your heart and move your will.

You will also discover her love for priests and vocations and her truly contemplative soul. Maybe you also will be moved to ask for her help as you pray for vocations and for the priests who serve you.

I am sure you will enjoy reading about Audrey, and I am also sure that something in this book will change you.

Father Anthony Bannon, LC
Cheshire, Connecticut, April 2008

INTRODUCTION

Le Châtelard, Les Avants sur Montreux,
Switzerland, April 1996

The snow crunched under my feet as I walked outside to the ground floor door. I pulled my overcoat around me and hid my nose in a scratchy Scottish scarf. There was the white and solitary statue of Mother Mary, and the big pine tree, its tired arms bending under the burden of snow. The path led behind a Nordic chapel, the little church of Les Avants. Here we were. In the chalet, everything smelled like home. I climbed up the creaky stairs into the sunny living room. Through the windows, one could catch a glimpse of blue down below: Lake Léman. Sometimes it was covered by a blanket of clouds; sometimes it seemed as if one was flying—blue sky above, white sky below.

I got settled in the dining room with an elementary tape recorder and a yellow cassette. Sunlight filled the room, lighting up the tablecloth with its white and blue squares. Beatrice was prancing about shoeless with her socks on crooked, while Lillian heated up some water for tea, which she served in a bowl, Swiss style. The tape recorder seemed to be broken, so we ended up using a plastic one the children proudly produced. That's how everything began.

I had few memories of Audrey. Yes, there was that day in Rome. I came out of the Giustiniana Center to go to the Aurelia Seminary with a French family that was spending Christmas in our guesthouse. In the car, I rode in the backseat with the girls. Such a blond family! One of the girls, more blond than the others, sat on my lap. Looking back, I realized that it was Audrey.

One day, after a taping session, Beatrice stood in my way on the stairs. She playfully hugged my legs and asked, "Why are you writing a book about my sister?"

I still haven't answered that question. It might be that someone gave Audrey the idea. Or it might be all hers. But this time, I didn't go out to look for her; it was she who came to me. And she hasn't left me in peace until she has said all that she had to say.

This book is not her biography, nor is it a kind of eulogy. It would be much better if whoever reads it finds himself simply with her, with the story told from her Mummy's mouth. Nothing more; nothing less. A flower needs no more adornment than what it has received from its Creator; everyone can see what inspires its beauty.

CHAPTER I

❦

childhood signs

"Here is the Master that I give you. He will teach you all that you have to do. I want you to read in the book of life, in which is enclosed the science of LOVE."

WORDS OF CHRIST TO ST. MARGARET MARY OF ALACOQUE, CITED BY ST. THÉRÈSE OF LISIEUX

"Children, as they grow in wisdom, stature, and grace before God and men, will be a precious help for the edification of the family community and for the sanctification of their own parents."

JOHN PAUL II, FAMILIARIS CONSORTIO

A Little Girl is Born

Audrey was born in Paris on March 18, 1983. Everything went well during the great event, although as we know, anything can happen in childbirth. Or, rather, exactly what has to happen happens. In the middle of the night, Lillian felt the baby coming, and coming quickly. In the midst of her nervousness and pain, she found it nearly impossible to awaken her husband, Jerome. Finally, she managed to wake him up, only to watch him search desperately for the missing car keys. They ended up taking a taxi—luckily, at that hour the streets were almost deserted—and they arrived with twenty minutes to spare.

This baby girl was very different from her big sister Aline. Among other things, she was born with a lot of hair, and black hair at that.

Jerome and Lillian organized the baptism right away. Lillian's parents lived in the United States and had come to Paris for a few days, so they wanted to take advantage of the opportune moment. They chose the 23rd of April for the christening.

The young couple lived in Paris, on rue Léon Cogniet[1], right next to Park Monceau. They went to the Church of St. Charles of Monceau, the parish closest to them. To get ready for the baptism they just had to dress up nicely, put the little girl in her baptismal clothes, prepare the home for an elegant cocktail party following the ceremony, invite their friends and families, and everything would be all set. Prepare spiritually for the baptism of a daughter? Go talk to a priest? Lillian hadn't thought of that. In those days, Lillian attended Sunday Mass but, like many other people, she didn't think of doing anything more. Certainly, for Lillian, the baptism was important and had to be done, even though she wasn't fully aware of what it meant. And it occurred to her to invite Marc, her husband's twin brother, to baptize his

---

1. "Rue" is the French word for street.

one-year-old child together with Audrey. At that time, Marc and his wife were not practicing Catholics, but they did accept the idea.

Presiding over the ceremony was a visiting African priest. In the homily, before the audience of Sunday Catholics, he declared, "Who knows if the Lord will call one of these children to the religious life?" Upon hearing those words, four-week-old Audrey gave a squeak, as if he had "hit the mark," provoking not a few meaningful chuckles and smiles among the grandparents. The incident was forgotten shortly afterwards among the greetings, the glasses of champagne, and the canapés served on silver trays. Such is life.

I will go to "caramel"

Three years later, the whole family was spending their summer vacation in Normandy. By that time one more child had been born, Henry. An enchanting little boy with a blond head full of curls, he was carried in his father's arms.

The family visited Lisieux, the city of St. Thérèse of the Child Jesus, and Les Buissonets, her home as a young girl. It was an enjoyable visit for all. Aline, five years old, her hair in braids and her hands stuck to the glass display windows, was intent on examining the museum exhibit of toys that St. Thérèse had played with as a girl. A recording for tourists told the life of St. Thérèse. Audrey was very quiet; even at age three, she was observing everything, listening with her eyes wide open, looking at this and that. Her little hands reached out to touch the bedspread, the curtains, the locks on the doors.

"Audrey, we only touch with our eyes," Mummy reminded her gently.

Immediately, she withdrew her hands as if something had burned them. A little later, the girls strolled about in the garden of Les Buissonets. In the middle, among immaculate hedges and little benches bordered by multicolored flowers, there stood a bright white sculpture representing St. Thérèse's father seated on a bench, with his beard and his pocket watch, while young Thérèse, her hair gathered in a bow, sat at his side, hands clasped together. She was begging him, "Papa, I want to enter Carmel!"

Upon leaving St. Thérèse's house, the family walked a few blocks to the Carmel convent in which St. Thérèse spent much of her life. They didn't see much in the museum, but they did note the dark brown habit that the saint wore and the beautiful cascade of light brown curls that had been cropped off upon her taking the veil.

On their return home, in the car, Audrey announced, "When I am grown up, I will go to *Caramel*." With her sweet tooth, "caramel" was a word she knew well!

In The confessional

A few months afterwards, back in Paris, Lillian brought the children to Mass. She entered the church, taking care that they didn't make too much noise, and sat down in a pew in the middle, holding Henry in her arms. She was uncomfortable, because their fourth child was on the way. A few moments later, Audrey got up from her seat and took Henry, who was just beginning to walk, to the back of the church. *Just what I need,* Lillian groaned to herself. *If I get up in my state, I'll just call attention to us.*

Henry appeared after a little while, and she immediately brought him to her side, but Audrey seemed to have disappeared. When Mass ended, Lillian went to the back of the church to get her daughter, trying to give herself reasons not to be angry: "She's just a little girl…" She found Audrey seated comfortably inside a confessional. The youngster jumped up from the kneeler, shook out her dress, and skipped over to her mother.

"Audrey, what were you doing? I didn't know where you were."

With wide eyes full of wonder, Audrey replied, "Mummy, there was a cross in there with Jesus on it. Just looking at him, you love him."

Lillian was taken aback. She felt a little frightened. *What did the child mean? Where has she gotten all this?* she thought. For the first time, she saw a previously unknown dimension of her daughter, a sacred dimension that went beyond her.

Montmartre

That year, Aline joined a group called "The Child Adorers of Montmartre." Once a month, some fifty children went with their young mothers to the Sacred Heart Basilica to adore the Blessed Sacrament. From 1870 onward, the citizens of Paris have had the privilege of perpetual adoration of the Eucharist, which is solemnly exposed in the basilica that majestically dominates the city from the top of a hill. Normally, very few people go there. It is dark and empty, and that huge tabernacle is all alone. But on the day the children go, it's like a big party. Lillian didn't bring her children there out of an excessive love for prayer, but because it was a lively group, a new group with the right sort of people.

The children stayed for half an hour before Jesus in the Eucharist. The prayers were adapted to their age, and between the songs, the lights, and the commotion of the children and their mothers, there wasn't even a minute of boredom.

Three-year-old Audrey had vehemently refused to stay in the nursery while her older sister went to such an interesting place. She sat at her sister's side and participated in all of the activities with dedication and enthusiasm, behaving beautifully, as some small children do when they sense the importance of the moment. She attracted attention because of her small size and her attentive concentration. She already had a very clear awareness of the real presence of Christ in the Eucharist. She gazed around with her big blue eyes at the grown-ups who were telling the children where they had to go, when they had to kneel, and how they should make their genuflection. A priest pointed to the tabernacle, saying gently, "This is Jesus, and he listens to everything that you want to tell him." Audrey drank in those words with her eyes.

There are people who cannot forget the perfection with which she made religious gestures. That careful way of making the sign of the cross, that characteristic smile.... She seemed so tiny in the procession line, moving forward so ceremoniously and seriously down the nave of the great basilica, with her arms crossed over her chest to receive a blessing. She did everything with the greatest solemnity, as if she were doing it before the very court of heaven. Next to her, it would have looked unseemly to sit with one's legs crossed or greet a friend too effusively. Without intending to, this little girl, hardly three feet tall, was already becoming an open book of lessons for those around her.

when the essential is missing

Lillian was overwhelmed. She didn't know where to start. There were boxes all over the place, lamps wrapped in parcel paper, sawdust and wood shavings, electrical cables on the floor, disassembled beds, rolled up rugs...and Jerome, her husband, was not there. He had rushed off to help prepare a Family Congress. The Billings couple would be there, as well as Mercedes Wilson and Mother Teresa of Calcutta. The event was fast approaching. But they hadn't been able to postpone the move, and today was a day of tying up loose ends. Lillian told herself that she simply had to get through it without losing her calm or her energy. Meanwhile, the children were running all over the new apartment, whose empty rooms seemed to magnify the sound of their shouts and laughter. Long hallways are wonderful for skating in socks, and the empty boxes were a forest of opportunities for climbing up and down, jumping in and out, hiding....

"Children, come here! Wouldn't you like to help Mummy a bit?"

Aline obediently set about carrying the boxes labeled "toys" to what would be her room. Audrey cast a glance around and said, very decisively, "Mummy, we're missing the most important thing." Henry, already a year old, was seated in his little chair, contemplating the scene and teething on his blanket. There was a moment of silence. Lillian, grateful for the quiet, began ordering the work in her head, unpacking, planning, and looking around at her new home: the light coming in here, a plant there, the color of the curtains, a spot for a small couch....

"Well, just think that we have a home! Little by little, we'll start putting everything in its place."

Audrey had disappeared. She came back after a good hour and asked, "Mummy, will you give me some tape, please?"

Lillian gave it to her without asking what it was for. A minute later, she saw Audrey on her tiptoes, sticking something to the wall just above the fireplace. When Audrey had finished the operation, she ran out of the room. Curious, Lillian came closer and examined the new decoration. Was it a drawing? It was something on paper. Ah! It was a paper crucifix painstakingly cut out, a drawing of Jesus crucified. True, it was more of an insinuation than a drawing by this three-year-old artist, but nevertheless, it was recognizable with his pink-colored body, the crown of thorns, and some red rays of blood. Lillian smiled wryly to herself. *These children!* She continued her work. As she went from room to room, she discovered paper crosses everywhere. *So it wasn't just for the living room!* Audrey had put a cross in every room: in the kitchen, in the laundry room, in the small guest bathroom, in the hallway.

Two days went by, and the house began to take shape. The crosses stayed taped on the wall. It hadn't occurred to anyone to remove a single one. Audrey had put them up! Sometime later, when the house was ready to receive guests, a friend came over for dinner. He thanked them later with a card, without failing to mention (with great discretion) his surprise to see an apartment so beautiful and elegant, with that fireplace, the mirrors, and the curtains—yet invaded everywhere by little paper crosses.

pencils in shoes

One day Lillian was coming back with Audrey from school. They were ten minutes from the house and traveling on foot, as they always did. It was March, and the little girl had just turned four. Lillian always picked up her children at midday to bring them home for lunch. Over time Audrey had acquired the custom of asking her mother for the keys to the apartment and running ahead to get into the house first. She wanted to have the table all set for Mummy before her arrival. It pleased Audrey so much to make this tender little gesture that Lillian felt she couldn't set the table before going to the school, in order to leave it for her daughter to do. But today, on their walk home, Audrey didn't go off running, and Lillian noticed that she was having difficulty walking.

"What's wrong, Audrey?"

"Nothing."

Lillian thought, *She put her shoes on wrong.* They stopped for a moment on the sidewalk.

"Let's see, Audrey. What do you have in your shoe?"

Audrey, leaning on her mother, obediently lifted her foot. Lillian, bending down, unbuckled the shoe and took it off. Some small colored pencils fell out. Audrey looked at her mother and said innocently, "It's because that way I don't have to carry them in my hand." Lillian looked at her, unconvinced. "Mummy, that's how I resist."

She had never heard Audrey say anything like this before. After this incident, Lillian, a little worried, began to observe her daughter more closely. She realized that Audrey was offering things to Jesus, and she tried to remember whether at some time she had told Audrey about things that saints did. How did she get this in her head? Actually, Lillian had been very careful not to tell her children about sacrifices, and she refrained from telling them saint stories that might make too much of an impression on their imaginations. She was looking for a spiritual development for her children that would be as healthy, spontaneous, and positive as possible. No strange things. No exaggerations. But Audrey started to say "I resist" so often that it was becoming second nature to her. And she said it smiling, without fussing, when it was extremely cold on the way home from school, when she was making a great effort carrying games and books from one side of the house to the other, or when one of her siblings wanted to go first.... Where had she gotten that?

Everyone in the house soon noticed Audrey's "enthusiasm" for offering little things to Jesus. Jerome was the first to recognize that, in a family of five small children, it is very practical when one of the children sacrifices her likings for the others. It simplified life enormously, especially when there wasn't enough white meat on the chicken to go around and "someone" had to take dark, or when they had burnt a piece of toast, or when Mummy insisted they finish off the last, little remaining bit and nobody wanted it. In this family, that "someone" was Audrey, in a systematic way. She would take the cake from the kitchen to the table, and the other children, exclaiming excitedly, would stretch out their plates, running to get the first piece. Audrey would move to the other end of the table, as if the cake didn't interest her very much. If she got some, she got some. If not, well, that was fine. And Lillian went from asking Audrey, "Are you sure you don't want any more cake?" to automatically letting her go without seconds. She had to force herself to remember that, in reality, Audrey loved cake just as much as anybody else. But Lillian had become so used to Audrey denying herself that it began to seem normal. And of course, it also became normal that Audrey never allowed any other member of the family to make "the effort." How one forges oneself!

And did Audrey ever love to eat! Shrimp cocktail in avocado halves, French fries, and most especially, chocolate mousse. Her eyes would shine, and she would squirm around in her chair when Mummy put it on the table. When she went with her Granny, Lillian's mother, to buy candies, she would gaze anxiously at the shop window and tell her, "The hardest thing is to save up." Then she would confess her big worry: "Granny, I think I am a bit greedy."

Audrey always thought of others. Once, she arrived home from a birthday party all pink, disheveled, and weighed down with candies. Upon entering the house, she greeted everyone in passing and went directly to the dining room table as if she had something extremely important to do. She then spilled her booty and divided all the sweets into equal piles. With her face full of excitement, she imagined how happy each one would be to receive such a wonderful gift. She was incapable of eating her candies without sharing them with her brothers and sisters. For them, Audrey was like a kind of Santa Claus. No one in the house was capable of acquiring such quantities of good things. Then, naturally, came the distribution. What was hers was everyone's.

On some occasions, she carried it to extremes. She was hardly four-and-a-half years old when she carried out an eminently Franciscan[2] gesture. One day, Lillian was looking for a sweater for Audrey. She entered Audrey's room and opened her dresser drawer. It was completely empty.

"What is going on?"

Aline's drawer, on the other hand, was stuffed to the brim. After much effort, they managed to pry it open. My, oh my! Audrey had forced all of her clothes into her sister's drawer. Aline had already seen it and had thought that it was crazy. But she hadn't said anything, thinking that if Audrey had done it, she had a reason.

Lillian asked Audrey, "What have you been doing?" Audrey responded with great determination: "I have decided to be poor, and I am going to keep only what I am wearing now."

lost in the park

Audrey loved her American grandparents, Lillian's parents, very much. She saw them less often than her paternal grandparents, who lived in Paris all year long. Grandpa came from the United States for a visit when Grégoire, the fourth child, was about to be born. He got along marvelously with his little granddaughter Audrey. His seriousness was a little intimidating to the other grandchildren, and they didn't dare be too effusive with their grandfather, so as not to bother him. But Audrey was different. She threw herself into his arms, smiled at him, joked with him, played with him as with any other member of the family, and Grandpa was very thankful for such displays of trust.

One day, he took her for a walk to the park, which was ten minutes from the house on rue Jouffroy, past Péreire Boulevard

---

2. As a young man, St. Francis gave away all of his possessions and joyfully embraced poverty for love of Christ.

and across the bridge over the many tracks of the St. Lazare train station. It was a small park called les Batignolles, a peaceful, shady garden. Leafy trees, not too high, narrow paths, thick hedges, a pond with a little waterfall, and a bit of sand for the children to play in with their buckets, their shovels, their trucks, and their balls. Here and there one would see young pregnant women, mothers with their baby carriages, and some *au pair* girls taking care of the little ones. An old gentleman sat reading a newspaper on a dark green bench, while further on a man sold balloons, and hundreds of birds trilled ceaselessly. It was a pretty park, a real park.

Grandfather and granddaughter enjoyed the beauty together. Audrey darted about everywhere, exploring. But in one of her expeditions, Grandpa lost sight of his little one. It happened so quickly! He retraced his steps, calling to her over and over, his voice growing deeper and more anguished. It was impossible to find her among so many children, with the sun flashing through the trees and among the intricate pathways and the many hedges.

At home, the doorbell rang. Lillian opened the door and saw Audrey's tiny figure. She was very flushed, panting for breath, but overflowing with light and joy. She ran inside.

"Well, Audrey, what are you doing?"

"Here I am!" she said, triumphantly.

Lillian thought that she had raced her grandfather home, and that he must be just behind her on the stairs. At that moment, the phone rang.

"Lillian! I've lost Audrey—she disappeared from my sight, and I can't find her!" It was Grandpa, deeply worried.

"But Dad, Audrey is here with me. She just arrived."

"What? That's impossible! How did she get home by herself? You don't know what the traffic is like out here. She would have had to cross the bridge with all those traffic lights, the cars and the buses, and then find the crosswalk at the boulevard traffic light!"

Lillian was alarmed. Her father was right. Audrey didn't know which street to take. Before getting to rue Jouffroy, she would have had to cross the rue de Saussure and the rue des Fermiers. And how would she have found the house? During the Napoleon III epoch, the architect Haussman had designed the type of buildings that have given Paris its distinctive style, but those buildings have a particular characteristic: they all look the same.

"Audrey, come here and tell me what happened."

Audrey was breathing normally now, and her face was still full of smiles, delight, and happiness. With the little voice of a four-year-old girl, she explained to her mother, "I got lost, so then I went to a lady and told her that I was lost. She told me to go to the police station."

(Surely, the lady gave her a complicated explanation of how to get there.)

"Then I prayed to my Guardian Angel and ran straight after Jesus."[3]

The consolation

Around this time, a statue of the Virgin Mary in Japan weeping blood caused quite a stir. Lillian was listening to a tape about the Virgin of Akita and had put it on in her room while resting because she didn't want the children to hear it. But Audrey asked her, "What is that?" so Lillian explained, "It's the Blessed Virgin who cries because the sins of men make her very sad."

A few days later, Lillian found Audrey on her knees in the hallway. She was kneeling in front of an image of our Lady where

---

3. J'ai demandé a mon Ange Gardien et j'ai couru tout droit en suivant Jésus.

the family gathered for a simple prayer every night before going to bed. She was there alone looking at Mary, looking at the flowers in front of the image, and very quiet.

"What are you doing, Audrey?"

"I'm consoling her."

She repeated this procedure on many other occasions. Between games and running about, she would put herself there on her knees for a good while, without warning. And her brothers and sisters would continue playing, running, and shouting. Jerome came and went without paying attention; it was a place of passage. It became normal to see her there. That was Audrey.

"Where is Audrey?"

"Over there, saying her prayers…."

Sometimes she stayed just a little while; on other occasions, longer. And at any given moment, she would decide that that was enough, and one would hear her say out loud, "That's enough. She's not crying anymore." And then she would go play.

My friend, saint Jude

Audrey's best friend was Saint Jude. In France, when one wants to find a lost object, one prays to Saint Anthony. In the United States, it's Saint Jude. Lillian knew this and prayed to him from time to time when she had lost something. Audrey heard her one day and took it to heart, to the point of creating a real partnership between herself and Saint Jude. Before long, everyone in the house had the habit of asking Audrey to pray to her friend Saint Jude whenever something was lost in order to find it again. And it would appear, surprisingly. It was a great advantage in this household, since they frequently tended to lose things: car keys, Mummy's pen, Papa's socks, the baby's bib, etc.

"Audrey, quick! Tell your friend to help us find the keys, or we'll be late!"

"Fantastic! I have them in my coat pocket."

It worked, even though they didn't really believe Saint Jude was responsible for recovering the items. Nevertheless, they liked the idea so much that it became kind of a joke among the family. When family friends came over for dinner, they talked about it.

"In this house, it's automatic—when you lose your wallet, you tell Audrey, 'Have Saint Jude find it,' and *voila!* In a jiffy, you have your wallet in your hand."

But Audrey would concentrate and pray to Saint Jude with all her strength. The little girl was truly convinced that the lost item was going to show up. On one occasion, Henry's christening medal was lost while the children were playing a game. The whole family searched for it. Suddenly, it reappeared, exactly where they had all been looking. Lillian had the strange sensation that it had been moved just so it could be found. But, even then, they still didn't manage to believe in it—at least, not like Audrey believed.

One day, when Audrey was five, she received a personal visit from her friend Saint Jude. It was a Friday, and she had come home from school in the mid-afternoon. Upon entering the house, she left her book bag on the floor and went running to play with Aline. Lillian picked up the book bag from the entryway, took out that week's dirty school smock, and tossed it on the laundry pile. Ten minutes later, Audrey appeared in the entryway. She had remembered that she needed to put her smock in the wash so that it would be clean for Monday. Oh, but it wasn't in her book bag where she had put it! After looking everywhere, her next step was to ask her friend Saint Jude, "Where is my smock?"

Audrey raced into the kitchen. She was beaming, as if something marvelous had happened to her. She held the smock in her hands.

"Mummy, I couldn't find my smock, so I prayed to Saint Jude and he led me to it! I found it in the laundry basket."

That day, for Audrey, the spiritual world in which she believed had come intensely close. Her mother asked her innocently, "And did you say thank you to Saint Jude?" The little girl responded enthusiastically: "Oh yes, I covered him with kisses!"

shepherded by a lamb

It was lunchtime and everyone was sitting around the table. Lillian began serving the little ones first.

"In this family, it would be good if we said grace," Audrey declared.

Aline looked at Papa. Papa looked at Mummy, who returned his gaze. Jerome and the others stood up, and he improvised a prayer of blessing. Then they sat down as if nothing had happened. To this very day, the family stands and says grace before every meal.

It was her special talent, Audrey's particular knack. She knew how to make certain decisions for the whole family, and it wouldn't occur to anybody to disagree—like that day when, in a simple comment, she told her parents, "It would be more elegant if we spoke to you using the *"vous"* form." (In France it is still a custom in traditional families with good manners for the children to address their parents and grandparents using the more formal *"vous"* instead of the more familiar *"tu."*) And so it was. Aline, Henry, Grégoire, and then Beatrice—that is, all of Audrey's brothers and sisters—began to speak to Jerome and Lillian using *"vous,"* and without the least bit of distance in their family relationships. Nobody put forth a single objection to the initiative.

Little by little, Jerome and Lillian began to let themselves be influenced by the special signs of goodness that Audrey left in her wake. In their little daughter, there was developing—almost imperceptibly—an instinct towards the highest perfection, a great refinement and delicacy towards others, and a deep sense of the sacred.

On one occasion, some close friends invited Lillian and the girls to a birthday party for one of their young nieces, Pauline, who had Down syndrome. Lillian accepted the invitation with pleasure, although she had to brace herself a bit for the uncertain nature of the party. It was the first time that Aline and Audrey were going to see a child with Down syndrome. Lillian thought to herself, *I hope my girls will behave well and not make any inappropriate comments about Pauline; let's hope they don't ask questions or stare at her. Well, we'll see how it goes.*

The party went fine, and the girls maintained their composure, thanks be to God. They came back home on foot. Deep down, Lillian was relieved. Suddenly, Audrey, who had just turned four, told her, "I really liked going to Pauline's house because she opens my heart." Lillian was surprised, but said nothing. A little further on, Audrey spoke up again. "Pauline is like Rose." (Her aunt Rose, Lillian's sister, was also handicapped). "You can tell that Jesus loves them very much."

Lillian realized then how much Audrey had understood: everything. Little by little, she was discovering the sense of the sacred that her daughter had been mysteriously acquiring.

Another time, when Audrey was still four, they were all together attending Mass on the night of the Easter Vigil. It was a long Mass, and very tiring, especially for a child. During the celebration, Audrey unexpectedly lost a baby tooth. We all know the impact that this event has on a child. Normally, it gives rise to a whole avalanche of sensations and expectations: the new smile, the new future teeth, jokes about the big gap, etc. But

Audrey must have thought that this was neither the time nor the place to make a scene. Without saying a word, she quietly put the tooth in her pocket. Lillian didn't realize anything had happened until, on the way home, Audrey announced, "Look, I lost a tooth!"

Around Christmas of that same year, Lillian stepped out of the house to go for a walk with her two girls. They were going to see the shop windows of the big Parisian department stores. The windows were beautifully decorated, with moving dolls and lights—a dream for girls of that age. They had to brave the cold December wind and the press of the crowds, but off they went. Before arriving at the shop windows, they passed two tramps who were sleeping in the street, curled up on pieces of cardboard over a grid in the sidewalk where warm air from the subway came up. Audrey stopped suddenly and stood looking at them intently. Lillian tried to steer her daughter away, saying, "Let's go, Audrey." Lillian had told her children about poor people, to teach them and to make them realize that poverty existed in the world, even though one didn't see it too much in Paris.

As Lillian prompted the girls to walk along, Audrey asked, "Mummy, why are they there? Can't we take them home?"

Lillian responded, "I don't think so, Audrey. You see—it's a little complicated." Lillian tried to explain why it wouldn't be best to bring these people into their home.

But Audrey objected, "But the apartment is very big, and I could sleep on the floor and they could sleep in my room." It was impossible to get the idea out of her head. She already had it all figured out. There was no way in Audrey's mind that those poor men should sleep out on the sidewalk in the cold.

Lillian could feel herself becoming frustrated, as she tried in vain to convince her daughter. It went far beyond common sense. In the end, the whole incident became a big drama, and because of it, the shop windows, the dolls, and the lights became an empty show. Aline was disillusioned, Audrey was indignant, Mummy was tired, and that's how they returned home. The gay little outing was ruined. Upon arrival: dinner and bed. Audrey said nothing more to her mother, but maintained a severe, penetrating look until she went to bed. As for Lillian, she would never forget. It was as if Audrey were telling her, "Mummy, you are not the least bit charitable."

During the Family Congress in September of 1986, Jerome and Lillian got to know Father Pierre, a Catholic priest who belonged to a religious order called the Legionaries of Christ, and they began to follow a path of greater growth in their Christian life. One morning, Lillian went for spiritual direction, and Father Pierre recommended that she dedicate some time to prayer first thing in the morning. Lillian tried to convince Father that this was impossible. The early hours were spent amidst the baby's crying, the feeding bottle, the diapers, making breakfast for the family, getting the children ready for school, and seeing her husband off to work. One had to be realistic. There was no way she could just close herself in a room to pray and let the children get themselves ready for the day. On the way back home, she went over the conversation in her mind. "Men just don't realize what it means to be a mother…" That same day, upon arriving home from school, Audrey told Lillian, "Mummy, I was thinking that I could make breakfast for the little ones in the morning so that you can have a little moment with Jesus." Audrey knew nothing about Lillian's appointment that morning, nor did she know what they had discussed. Lillian was astounded.

These events sometimes caused tensions between the family and their friends because the family's customs became so unconventional. They were often told, "But you are the ones who have to educate that child—she is not in charge of you!" to which Jerome and Lillian would respond: "The problem is that she's right."

At this time, Aline began participating in the activities of the Theresian Mission (*Mission Thérèsienne*). This was a movement organized by a diocesan priest named Father Thévenin. It consisted of teaching and motivating children to pray for vocations. Each of the older children would spiritually adopt a priest and commit themselves to praying for him every day. The children received a paper poster with a quite lengthy prayer for priests printed on it. As soon as Audrey heard Father Thévenin's explanation about the mission of the children as guardians of priestly vocations, and as soon as Aline received her prayer for priests, she hung the prayer poster in the hallway at home, next to the Virgin Mary, so that she could pray it every night.

When Lillian saw this bright, apple-green sheet of paper hanging in the front hall, she agreed to say the prayer, but she was not at all pleased about its prominent position, right near the entry to the house and in full view of everyone. It was such an ugly shade of green! Audrey was the first to learn it by heart, and her parents are convinced that she prayed it every day for the rest of her life. This prayer planted in her soul one of the principal seeds of her spirituality: love and zeal for vocations, especially for priests.

First Holy Communion

Jerome and Lillian were a young couple with five small children who were just as noisy and mischievous as the rest. Until a short while ago, their religious practice had consisted of Sunday Mass and little else. Nevertheless, they realized that they did have a problem, or a challenge, or a mystery: their daughter Audrey. By now, her spirituality had gone way beyond what one could consider "normal." They saw it clearly; it was obvious. They worried, but they didn't know what to do.

After an evening at the theater with their good friends Caroline and Omer, they went out for a drink and mentioned a few of their worries. "Audrey bewilders us; she is beyond us. We don't know what to do with her. We don't understand where to go."

A few days before, Lillian had told Jerome, "Audrey seems to know her catechism without anyone having taught it to her. She just understands the mysteries of the faith. It is as if they aren't mysteries for her." They had the sense that someone at home was teaching Audrey without their knowledge, although nobody was. And it isn't so pleasant for parents to feel that their five-year-old daughter is "going her own way."

One night, they invited Father Pierre, whom they already considered a close friend of the family, to come over for dinner. They asked him, "What should we do with Audrey? How should we teach her?" The priest limited himself to saying, "Don't do anything. Follow her." This advice took root in their minds and hearts during the weeks, months, and years to come. It became their way of handling not only Audrey but also their other children.

Audrey wanted to receive her first holy Communion. And she wanted to do it on the fifteenth of August of that year, the closing day of the Marian Year, a year specially devoted to Mary. In addition, she wanted to do it in Lourdes. The family had made a short visit there the year before. In France, children normally make their first communion at age nine or ten with their catechism class in the parish. Audrey was only five. Her parents asked Father Pierre: "And now what do we do? Do we just 'follow her'?"

The priest wanted to be sure that the girl's motives were deep ones, that she was sure she wanted it, so he put some obstacles in her way. First, she had to obtain the approval of a diocesan priest, and after that, approval from another priest. Audrey lent herself to the good Fathers' inquiries with docility, but her mother could tell that she considered it quite unnecessary and was only doing it to humor them.

At last, the day arrived: August 15, 1988, the day of the closing of the Marian Year. Lourdes was packed with people. They swarmed around the grotto and the basilica and made the area an anthill of banners, flags, hats, and uniforms from the boy scouts, the Red Cross, and a thousand confraternities, movements, and pious associations. There were endless lines of people with illnesses waiting in wheelchairs for their turn between the songs and invocations to pray in the grotto. It was the day of France's national pilgrimage and a solemn Marian feast day. The holy Marian Year had come to an end, and on that day everything was an expression of thanksgiving to the Blessed Mother. Finally, the family found a quiet little corner to have the simple ceremony. It would be in the little chapel of St. Michael, in the crypt just above the grotto.

Father Pierre had sensed in Audrey an intense desire to receive Jesus, and he was the one who placed the Body of Jesus on her lips for the first time. Smiles appeared on the faces of the tourists who happened to see such a little girl wearing a crown of flowers and happily walking about in her white first holy Communion dress. The dress, borrowed from a cousin, was the one Aline had worn for her first holy Communion a few months beforehand. But on Audrey it was far too big and nearly touched the ground.[4] No matter: Audrey marched radiantly along, leading the way through the crowds. She had succeeded in making her will prevail over everyone, and her parents watched her with growing wonder, asking themselves, "What is it about her?"

Little by little, her parents were discovering that there was an authentic love story between Audrey and Jesus, a love relationship of which they were the guardians and protectors.

---

4. Jerome and Lillian donated the dress to the Carmelite convent in El Escorial, Spain. The Mother Superior is the sister of their friend Father Ignacio Oriol, LC. It is displayed in the capitulary room there.

CHAPTER 2

# of flesh and blood...
and something more

"What does it mean that 'unless you change and become like children, you shall not enter the kingdom of heaven'? Is not Jesus pointing to children as models even for grown-ups? People who are destined to go to heaven are simple like children, and like children are full of trust, rich in goodness and pure."

— LETTER OF POPE JOHN PAUL II TO CHILDREN

how beautiful!

Audrey's first word was "beautiful" (*beau*). It seemed as if she was born to contemplate beauty. From the time she was very young, her eyes were always watching everything: intense, alert, full of wonder.

One day, Audrey went out alone into the garden. She was so young that she couldn't speak yet. Her gaze was fixed on the trees. As she tiptoed about here and there, she paid no attention to where she stepped; she was looking for the birds hidden in the branches and, reaching out for them with her little hands, she tried to imitate their sweet singing. She intently watched how they pecked at the ground. Then she discovered a nest— what a surprise! Her cheeks aflame with excitement, she went running to find Mummy. The discovery had filled the morning with delight.

Some years later, in the shady courtyard of her school, Louise de Bettignies, she would spend long moments squatting down, her hand extended towards the ground, her palms full of bread crumbs and her eyes fixed on the birds. She watched them advance and timidly retreat, and then come closer. One stretched out his beak, snatched a crumb, and then took flight. Before long, one of the pigeons came every day to eat out of Audrey's hand, without fear. It was her friend; she had tamed it. She named it "Coco."

She was crazy about flowers. After she turned three, her paternal grandparents often took her on outings, once to the Bagatelle Garden in the Bois de Boulogne. They remember their granddaughter's unique enthusiasm whenever she saw the beds of begonias, petunias, pansies, and roses in full bloom.

Audrey and her family spent their summers at Maillot, a house outside a small town in Normandy, close to Lisieux. There she could enjoy nature to the full. They remember that from a very young age there was one thing that caused her real heartache: a broken flower. She would walk into the house with it in her hands and cry an ocean of tears. And that would happen even though she usually didn't cry much. "But Audrey, it's no big deal!"

Her American grandmother taught her how to arrange bouquets of flowers. Audrey would sit on the front steps of the house and, with great care and concentration, arrange a bouquet for the middle of the dining room table.

In the mornings, she would enjoy immensely a walk in search of rabbits on the dairy farm next to Maillot. Afterwards, she would put peanuts in strategic places in the garden for the squirrels. And if she saw one, it wasn't long before everybody knew about it. Driving to the house with her grandfather, as the car would sweep up the drive, a little voice from the back of the car could predictably be heard: "Grampa, be careful of the little squirrel red."[1]

The days when she and Aline had horseback riding lessons were a real treat. Her pony was called Raspberry, and her young teacher had to "rein her in." "Audrey, when I teach you how to walk, you want to trot, and when I teach you how to trot, you want to gallop!" The little girl would laugh mischievously and look at her. (Actually, Aline knew that her sister greatly admired the teacher because of her hair: a lovely, free mane that went down to her waist.)

On vacation, Audrey loved to be active. She would gladly have spent the entire day bobbing in the pool, but the children weren't allowed to swim alone. In the morning, she would stroll in the garden, and then run to the cherry tree, which had a long branch from which she could hang and swing most marvelously. Audrey would hang and then let herself fall, yelling, "Tarzaaaaan!"

---

1. In French, the adjective is placed after the noun. At this age, Audrey still used the French grammatical order when she spoke English.

Afterwards, she would get together with her brothers and sisters on the tennis court, where they would chase each other on their bicycles until they were completely out of breath. After lunch came a veritable torture: naptime. Audrey wanted to jump in the pool, but she couldn't; first she had to wait an hour to digest her lunch. At the slightest gesture of permission from her mother, she would fly towards the pool. Her brothers and sisters, changing into their bathing suits, had barely gotten their socks off and she was already jumping into the pool with a shout of joy. The sound of Audrey's laughter in the pool…what laughter! It sounded like the tinkling of a little bell bubbling up from the bottom of her throat, making the others break into joyful laughter too.

When Lillian was expecting Beatrice, the fifth child, she discovered a water park near Paris. It had pools, water rides of all sizes, bridges, slides, and games. She took the children a few times. What a marvel! Lillian could sit on a *chaise longue* and let the children play from eight in the morning until eight at night. Audrey would spend the entire day jumping in and out of the water, running back and forth to her mother, never wanting the day to end. Audrey decided to call that place "Pleasure Island." Well, if you say so….

Drum

He was her dream: a black Labrador dog. They would name him Drum, and when he was old enough, they would all put on a circus show together with Audrey and Drum as the main attraction. Afterwards, she would go to Carmel. That's how she drew it one day on a sheet of paper: Audrey dressed in sequins with her magnificent dog, surrounded by a cheering crowd. At the bottom of the page, she wrote, "Continues." And on the next sheet: Audrey dressed as a Carmelite, her hands joined in prayer, with her rosary. A little girl's dreams….

At night, Lillian would tuck each one of her children into bed. "Another story, Mummy! Another kiss!" Typical children. It's difficult for a mother to try to leave the room.

Aline and Audrey slept in the same room, and they had it all planned out: they were in their pajamas, the light was off, and now they just had to wait. As Mummy's footsteps faded away down the hall…."Ta da!" The hour had come! They put on their school gym uniforms and pretended they were circus champions of the highest caliber, jumping from bed to bed in the half-light. Any little noise would be the end of everything.

"And now, ladies and gentlemen, Audrey and Drum!" Imaginary applause….

One night, Aline got a little annoyed and said, "Listen, it's *my* turn to be the main attraction," and the circus ended in tears and pouts. Back in bed again, the moment for a trick arrived. After a while, Aline heard Audrey fall out of bed in her sleep. Aline then got out of bed, picked up Audrey, and put her back in her bed. An explosion of laughter followed, and Audrey jumped up: "Fooled you, fooled you!"

Aline then went back to bed, and a little while later slipped to the floor as if she had fallen out of bed. Audrey responded, "I'm not fooled, Aline! You're just pretending!" Aline stayed on the floor for a long time, and it seemed like she didn't hear anything, so Audrey ended up believing that she really had fallen. Audrey picked up her sister and put her back in the bed. Aline tried to hide her laughter by pretending to be asleep and said nothing. The next day at breakfast, Audrey mentioned the incident and Aline pretended she didn't know anything about it. But inside, she was quite pleased and satisfied. This time, she had won.

A club at school

Aline was one grade ahead of Audrey at school, and she

hadn't made a lot of friends in her class. Audrey, on the other hand, was the ringleader of a little group of lively girls. At recess time, she would invite Aline to play with them so that she wouldn't feel left out.

One day, Audrey had the great idea of founding a club. To be a member, one had to be six or seven years old. Audrey organized everything: the president would be Aline since she was the oldest (note the tender detail towards her sister); the vice president would be Audrey's best friend; and all the rest would be associates. Behind the scenes, Audrey was the mastermind, heart, and leader of the group. She organized them, proposed games to play, and got them excited about playing…an intelligent way of guiding the group without imposing herself on any of her friends.

In Disguise

One of Audrey's favorite activities was to put on a disguise. Aline also had fun with disguises, but the sisters had very different tastes. Aline would finish getting ready in front of a mirror; one time she was a princess dressed in lace, her hair up, and wearing a crown and shiny shoes. Audrey, however, would wander about restlessly here and there, and then suddenly announce her disguise. One time she exclaimed, "That's it! I'm a Dalmatian!"

Quite pleased and satisfied, she set about greeting everyone, making funny faces and clownish antics in her bathing suit and bare feet, her hair disheveled, black spots painted all over her body and a big black snout, beneath which she had painted a smile.

But the most unforgettable incident was that birthday party when Audrey decided to disguise herself as an ugly old woman. She dressed in dark wool, wore a plaid shawl with a fringe, and gave herself a walking stick and a hunched back. She disheveled her hair and covered it with powder, and she put on a real witch's face—taking advantage of her missing teeth. Audrey was definitely in her element, enjoying herself immensely as she went about teasing her brothers and sisters with horrid cackles. One had to take advantage of these opportunities to the full.

A problem presented itself when the doorbell began to ring and the guests arrived. Lillian, who was very partial to freedom of expression, never imagined the fright that Audrey would give to her innocent and impeccable guests. "Oh, how horrible!" exclaimed one lady, while her little girl, dressed as an adorable pink fairy, clung to her skirt in terror.

More "cha-cha-cha"

Audrey always found a way to disguise herself, or at least to dress in her own style. Her disguises were original, and she had a very personal conception of what was in good taste. From a very young age, once she had learned, more or less, to dress herself, she would give herself the most incredible hairstyles. She had long, pretty blond hair. At the most unexpected moments, she would appear in the living room with her head full of all kinds of barrettes holding up little locks of hair in all different directions. They were red, yellow, gold, lacquered, and in the shape of butterflies. Audrey was quite pleased with herself: the more barrettes she had, the more beautiful she felt. Then she would complete the look with her clothes. With her hair pinned up, she would sally forth in an orange sweater, pink pants, and blue socks. Whatever she liked, she would put on, all at once.

Caroline, one of Mummy's friends, sometimes walked the girls to school in order to help Lillian. She and Aline felt quite embarrassed when they brought Audrey out on the street in her violet outfit covered with big pink tulips, sporting red and blue plaid socks and a head full of all kinds of barrettes. In Paris, little girls go to school perfectly dressed, with their smocked dresses, their little shoes buckled shut, and their hair cut short, parted on the side with a headband. But Lillian thought that it wasn't a bad idea to let Audrey dress herself as she pleased, without imposing a rigid style on her.

Mami, Audrey's paternal grandmother, came one day to pick her up at school. It was midwinter. "Audrey, how can you go out like that, with your legs bare in this cold?" Audrey had felt hot and had left the house with nothing covering her legs but a short skirt and shoes without socks.

When the girls were given the same clothes as gifts, invariably the blue would be for Aline and the red for Audrey. Aline always showed herself to be more sober, slender, and tranquil. Audrey, more round and attention-getting, was much more conscious of her "style." At home one day, with great freedom of spirit, she announced, "My sister Aline is a bit serious. I am more 'cha-cha-cha.'"

striving to be the best

Only our Lord could compose a perfect symphony combining uproar and silence, light and shadow, tropical colors and the tranquility of an Antarctic landscape. Audrey's soul had this richness of contrasts, and it made her a marvelous creature. Her joy was overflowing but not superficial. She was restless without being impatient, expressive but not extroverted, and she had authority without being bossy. From a young age, she knew how to distinguish between good and evil. She was conscious, lucidly conscious, with a sense of awareness unusual for her age. Audrey was adult in her awareness and wise in her knowledge of reality. She had a sense of the essentials. She seemed like a living compass, which at times was more than a little uncomfortable for some of her friends and her parents. Her needle pointed north (to God), as stubborn and firm as Nature herself. Without a doubt, this interior light was a gratuitous outpouring of the Holy Spirit, who sometimes makes himself present in children to remind us of our Lord's words: "I give you thanks, Father, Lord of heaven and earth, because you have hidden these things from the wise and the prudent, and have revealed them to merest children."[2]

Nevertheless, there was something that was extremely painful for Audrey: losing a game. For example, she loved to play "La Terre Promise" (The Promised Land) and would silently gear herself up to win. If she saw herself losing ground, she would get nervous. One day, in order to beat Audrey, Aunt Brigitte put herself on her older daughter Anne Sophie's team. Audrey noticed and became furious. Without saying a word, she seethed inwardly and her face showed her irritation. She let out a few sighs that seemed to say, "How ridiculous for you to try to beat me. I'm going to win without anyone's help." Audrey was one of those children who loved to organize her siblings and cousins, and they were always available to play. With great enthusiasm, she would hand out the chips, explain the rules, and give the signal to start. But when things became difficult and she saw herself starting to lose, she would lose her desire to play. This was evidence of her deep dislike of failure.

When she was seven years old, the whole family moved to La Celle St. Cloud.[3] Audrey resented this very much. Living in the city meant that one could have everything close by, go everywhere on foot, and go to a girls' school run by the Ursuline mothers (Louise de Bettignies), which she liked very much. Now they lived almost out in the country, in a house with a garden. They had to take the car to get anywhere.

The children changed schools after the spring break. The new school, Les Châtaigniers, was a small, coed school, more

---

2. Mt 11:25.

3. La Celle Saint Cloud is a residential area on the outskirts of Paris, near Versailles.

informal than their school in Paris. After a few weeks, Audrey began to feel restless. The grammar exercises in her new school were exactly the same ones she had done the year before at her old school, Louise de Bettignies. In fact, the old school was a year ahead. Even worse, since it was the middle of the year, they put her in a slower class with two levels, which meant she always had to wait for the younger ones to catch on. Audrey wanted to advance; she wanted to learn. She began to feel frustrated to the point of tears, and she lost her desire to go to school. "Mummy, I already know this. I'm not learning anything. Won't they put me in a higher class?"

It was not allowed. Audrey began to be disillusioned with her teachers; they were treating her like a little girl. She wanted to learn great things, and they didn't understand. Then she saw them during their breaks chatting about a thousand futilities and smoking together in little groups. With no challenges and no stimuli, she felt bound hand and foot. It's true that her relationships with the teachers in her old school had not always been easy, because in France it is not highly thought of for students to move a year ahead. Lillian had fought for it because she knew her daughter's capacity, but the teachers didn't think much of Audrey. They said, "This girl is very timid." Lillian tried to make them understand that if Audrey didn't talk much, it wasn't a matter of timidity, but of reserve. Nevertheless, the lack of encouragement from the teachers actually had a positive effect on Audrey, and instead of discouraging her, it spurred her on to a greater desire to learn and make progress. If they thought she could never meet the standards they set, she wanted to demonstrate that she could do even more. Leaving this challenging atmosphere accentuated her discouragement upon entering the Les Châtaigniers school.

Someone once said, "Not to demand that a loved one be the best is indifference, the opposite of love." Audrey understood that and suffered from it.

One morning, some young athletes came to the school to promote tennis classes. They were from the French Tennis Federation and were going to hold tryouts for children in order to detect future champions. Audrey came home in a state of great excitement. "Papa, let's go to the tryouts! I want to play tennis—I want to be a champion. Really, I can do it!" Her eyes were shining. She was totally convinced that she was going to become a star tennis player. She already saw herself crossing the court and hitting the ball in the championship game.

The day of the tryouts, she impatiently waited for her father in the living room, imitating the swing of the tennis players with imaginary racquet strokes in the air. On the way to the tryouts, she talked nonstop. Jerome smiled.

The court was right next to the school. They went on foot, in a sporty mood. Many mothers were there for the tryouts with their children. "Hi, Audrey!" It was her friends from school. Audrey felt nothing less than heroic. As the children went out onto the court two by two, Audrey looked on and repeated under her breath, "I'm going to get it, I'm going to get it." The little children were so cute with their racquets, which were almost as big as they were. Two young people from the French Tennis Federation were on one side of the net to test the children, watching their coordination, their agility, and their reflexes. Just by looking at the children, they were able to see if they passed the test or not. Next came Audrey's turn. She went out nervously, but decidedly, repeating to herself, "I'm going to get it." Jerome had known from the beginning that his daughter was not going to be chosen. Audrey came off the court serious, almost with tears in her eyes. The young trainers had given her encouragement, but she knew very well that she had not made it. They had told her in a nice way that they would call her with the results, but they clearly already knew the results. Jerome and Audrey walked back home. Audrey took her father's hand and didn't open her mouth the whole way there. She never spoke about tennis again.

It was hard to watch her high ideal of perfection clash head-on with her littleness. Audrey had to digest the hard lesson of not being able to meet all of her own expectations.

It happened again with the piano. Audrey and Aline were taking lessons. At the end of Audrey's first year, they had praised her to the skies after she had played a little piece in a simple recital. At home, her father told her, "Now play it for Mami." Beaming with pride and joy, she sat down at the keyboard to make her debut in front of her paternal grandmother. When she had finished, her father said to his mother, smiling, "Mami, now you play something." She, who had studied piano in the Paris Conservatory, sat down and played a simple but splendid piece by Mozart. Audrey's face grew pale and downcast. She had understood the message. Afterwards, the grandmother asked her son, "Why did you ask me to play? Poor child, look how it has affected her."

Jerome responded, "She has to realize that it takes a lot of work to get to perfection."

On the other hand, Audrey had learned to accept her physical appearance. She saw herself as ugly and laughed at herself, but she loved her long blond hair. She felt that it was the only thing about her that could shine.

What was really hard for her was to show her feet. One day, they went to the pediatrician's office for an examination, and the doctor told her that she had flat feet. Upon arriving home, Audrey was deeply annoyed and expressed her disagreement at dinner. "That doctor said I have flat feet." Everybody laughed, which annoyed her even more. In time, she resigned herself to wearing orthopedic boots and to the idea that she was not made perfect in every way. But on the day of her first Communion in Lourdes, she climbed up the stairs of the Rosary Basilica with great joy: not only was she fulfilling a dream, but she was also wearing beautiful, new, white shoes, like all the other girls.

Audrey was always grateful to have grandmothers who loved to see things done well: good manners, speaking properly, the thousand details of social forms, the elegant decoration of a home.... She would take all her questions to Granny, who delighted in giving detailed explanations to her granddaughter.

Audrey was interested in all the details of etiquette and manners. Regarding table manners, for example, she wanted to know whether one should keep one's hands on one's knees as they do in England, or if it was better to let them rest on the table, as in France. Her grandmother would sit down with her and try to remember everything she had learned from her French grandmother.

Audrey also loved to place the pastries on the table for teatime with utmost delicacy and perfection, and then consult her grandmother to see if she had done it well. She practiced making the sign of the cross with her, striving to do it perfectly. In the summer evenings after dinner, Granny taught her granddaughters how to knit. Audrey tried with all her might to make each stitch impeccable. If she made a mistake, she would undo it and start all over again.

It would Be More Elegant

Audrey's world was composed of things that were elegant and things that were not so elegant. Swearing was not elegant. Wearing miniskirts was not elegant. Smoking was not elegant. Using vulgar words was not elegant. And when something un-elegant was going on, Audrey refused to participate. She would take one look and then disappear. Her fine sense of correctness quickly detected subtle dissonances, which caused her pain and discomfort. And so she prayed that the others would become better.

One day, a friend of her parents came over for dinner. His vocabulary was not too polite, and Audrey did not approve. In France, sometimes certain swear words are used almost as a form of snobbery. Once the friend was gone, Audrey turned to her father and said very firmly, "I don't want that man to come over to our house ever again."

On another occasion, when Audrey was four, it happened that Aline innocently used a bad word at home. She hadn't realized it was wrong. Lillian corrected her: "I don't ever want to hear you say a word like that in this house."

"But Mummy," Aline replied, surprised, "at school, everyone says that."

"Well, that's very sad. The girls who say that at school aren't good friends for you."

"But that means we can't have any friends," protested Aline, "because everyone uses those words."

"In my class there is a boy who never says bad words," Audrey interjected. "His name is Pierre. He will be my only friend."

Birthday parties with schoolmates sometimes went badly. The other children fought, got dirty, used bad words, argued over prizes and candies, and took all the food. At one of these parties, Audrey burst into tears and had to be taken home. These assaults to her sensitivity were more than she could bear.

One day, she came home from school very sad. Almost no one in her class knew who Pope John Paul II was. And she had been so excited about him because she had been in Rome with her family during the Christmas holidays. She loved the Pope dearly and prayed daily for him and for his intentions. But another day was even worse. She began to cry because no one in the school knew who Father Pierre was. At home, she begged Lillian to make the school invite Father Pierre for a visit so that the nuns and students would get to know him.

The family got together every night to pray. In the entry hall of the apartment, there was a big mirror, and in front of the mirror, a small table with a statue of Our Lady. The children did their best to honor her with little flowers, drawings from school, holy cards, and pictures. They knelt down around the statue. On a door on the right, Audrey had put up the prayer for vocations that Father Thévenin had given her. It was that sheet of fluorescent green paper that Lillian disliked so much. Aline and Audrey would settle themselves in front and to the right. Audrey, with her hands together and her face very serious, would be very still. Jerome and Lillian would hold the little ones, who would usually start to squirm, sing loudly, start kicking, or touch Papa's face. "Un-elegant" things. Jerome would laugh at the scene and let the child continue. Audrey's gaze would turn tense, and she would fix her eyes on her father to the point of intimidation.

"Sorry, Audrey."

Audrey said so

Audrey, like any clever and lively girl, learned to speak at a young age. But the way she used the language drew attention. Those who knew her were immediately attracted by this little person whose childish voice spoke with such elegance and propriety. She spoke with an aristocratic accent, and yet with such sweetness and candor that there was not the least hint of pedantry in her speech. In her own way, she tried to express how much she loved those closest to her, and in her own way, she tried to find the best, most elegant, and most well-mannered way to say things.

"Mummy, may I have permission to leave this here?" "Mummy, may I see that photo, please?" "Papa, don't you think it would be more elegant if you stopped smoking?"

She made keen observations, and her verbal precision was capable of exposing anything. She was quick to sense and express the absurdity of a situation.

One day, when she was four, Audrey was coming home with her family from the beach on L'Ile de Re, in Brittany. Some friends were walking with them. From far off, they saw a woman crossing the beach and coming their way. This woman, of rather sizeable girth, was garishly dressed and laden down with bulky beach gear. She was pulling along her miniscule dog—one of those little "sausage dogs" whose paws go "tick-tick" on the sidewalk. Just as they crossed paths with the woman, Audrey exclaimed in a loud voice, "What a ridiculous little dog!" An explosion of laughter followed, and the poor lady, offended, accelerated her pace. The friends of Audrey's parents remarked on Audrey's gift for "hitting the nail on the head."

Perhaps something of the quality of her language came from her family. One of Jerome's grandfathers had been a professor at the Sorbonne. Her grandmother also had *le verbe facile*. Nevertheless, this quality in Audrey reinforced her maturity and authority. Maybe that was why her father was never able to deny her anything. Or maybe it was because Audrey was correct, both in what she said and in how she said it.

Since Audrey said so, they began to say grace before meals. Since she said so, the children spoke to the parents using the more formal *vous*. Since she said so, they prayed the prayer for vocations every day as a family. And since Audrey said so, the new baby was to be named Grégoire.

sometimes Little ones Teach Adults

Nevertheless, Audrey intimidated some people. She looked straight into one's eyes, and she had the ability to expose the soul, revealing a person's conscience to him. Some adults even commented to Audrey's parents that they felt uncomfortable being in front of Audrey. They said, "I don't know what it is about that girl, but she intimidates me." That was her power over adults. Without desiring it or insinuating anything, she became for them a kind of "sign of contradiction" because she "revealed the thoughts of many hearts." She was a little girl who didn't give her heart to just anybody; she was quite selective and reserved in her affections. Although she treated everyone with childlike kindness, she didn't give herself easily to just anyone. Her finely calibrated sensitivity could instinctively detect a lack of interior harmony in an adult. So she kept her distance and didn't respond effusively to the gestures of affection that these adults gave her. This sometimes produced a kind of frustration in some people close to the family, to the point that some considered her haughty and closed.

Jerome smoked a lot, which didn't please Audrey at all. She insisted, with great conviction, "Papa, it's not elegant to smoke. You must stop smoking; it's doing you harm."

"But what harm is there in smoking one little cigarette after a meal?"

These differences of opinion that were so common, for example, at the summer dinner table, were rather surprising to those who witnessed them. More than one would think, "But what business does this little girl have telling her father what to do?"

One day, Audrey's godmother Brigitte (Jerome's sister) went straight to the point. "Audrey, look. You're a little girl and your father is a grown-up. Why are you always telling him what he should and shouldn't do? It's not exactly normal. It's not correct."

Audrey merely wrinkled her nose. "It's for his own good."

They also asked Jerome why he let his daughter tell him what to do. He observed, "It's that, in the end, she's right." In reality, Jerome loved the way his daughter, his pearl, instructed him, for he felt a mixture of admiration and tenderness for her. Besides, his sensitive fatherly ear knew how to perceive the presence of God in his children.

Brigitte got along very well with Audrey. Sometimes they

spoke "woman to woman." One summer while they were together in Brittany, in La Baule, Brigitte took her goddaughter for an ice cream, just before Audrey and her family took the return trip to Normandy.

"Tomorrow you go back to Maillot, don't you?"

"Yes, and I'm worried," said Audrey. "Papa is tired and will have to drive for a long time. We're all going to end up in a ditch...."

Audrey missed nothing, and for this reason, she commanded respect. Odile, a friend of Lillian and Jerome's, will never forget one summer evening at Maillot. They had a summerhouse nearby, and their children played together. Odile and Audrey were busy playing "La Terre Promise" when Audrey looked up and quietly mentioned to Odile, in a most serious and discreet way, "Aimery has taken a caramel without your permission." Odile, a bit intimidated, had to admit that she had not kept very good watch over her son. She looked at her interlocutor for a moment and remembered watching her as she came down the stairs. Audrey went down in small steps, like little children do: first one foot, then the other—one stair. One foot, the other foot—next stair. At that moment, observing Audrey, Odile felt a shiver go down her spine. "She is small, so small; look at those little hands, her stature, her knees, her nose. And yet when she opens her mouth, she puts me in my place as if she were my own mother...."

Audrey had such authority because she had learned to obey before she learned to give orders. Lillian never had problems with her daughter in spite of Audrey's authoritarian character. Audrey was always docile to her mother's directions. Her mother would ask her for something and explain it, and Audrey would listen very attentively, with her big blue eyes wide open. She would understand it, and then go do it exactly as Mummy had said. It was enough for her simply to understand that something was good, and that it was a duty. She would then fulfill it completely, with conviction and right away. Lillian had to make sure that Audrey was not too unbending with her siblings, who were less prompt to obey.

She tended to take things very much to heart. One would see her come home from school and, without anybody saying anything to her, begin working on her homework with the utmost dedication. She worried if something didn't come out right or if she felt that she wasn't going to finish. It worried her to see Aline having difficulties finishing her homework.

There was something else that caught Lillian's attention early on: Audrey asked permission for everything, even when it wasn't strictly necessary. In their rooms, the children kept little bags of candy that they had received as gifts; it was normal to find one or another of them with a candy in their mouth. Before taking a candy from her bag, Audrey would come out of her room, find her mother, and ask her for permission to eat it. Lillian told her, "Of course you can take one. They're yours." Then Audrey would run back to her room.

On their first excursion to the water park (Audrey's "Pleasure Island"), there was a moment when Lillian no longer knew how she should act. She sat by the pool relaxing, relieved not to have to worry about the children for a while. The elder ones were off at the other end of the enormous pool, playing on inner tubes and going down slides into the water. She could hear the younger ones splashing in the shallow end, playing in the water. But here came Audrey running, soaking wet. She had just come out of the water after having been down a waterslide with her father.

"Mummy, Mummy, may I go again?"

"Yes, dear, of course. You're here to have fun; do whatever you want."

She ran back to go down the slide again. Every time she

wanted to go for another ride, she would come back running, full of joy and panting for breath, to ask Mummy for permission to go on the slide again. Then she would disappear, running off for another ride. Lillian was surprised and amused to note that Audrey, unlike the other children, would always rush back to her after going down the slide to ask permission to go again. Lillian considered telling her that she needn't bother, but she decided that it was probably safer and that she shouldn't discourage such spontaneous obedience. Truly, Audrey's parents, almost without realizing it, were learning many things from this little girl who was not yet six years old.

Brothers and sisters

One has to remember that Audrey's behavior was quite unlike that of her brothers and sisters. And this is not to say that her parents had educated her with a special emphasis on certain things. Jerome and Lillian knew how to create a family atmosphere where trust and freedom reigned so that each child could develop his or her personality in a free and natural way. Nevertheless, when it came to manners, Lillian did instill a great refinement in her children. On that point, she was quite strict with all of them. She demanded a lot from them in terms of respect, good manners, language, and good behavior with grown-ups. Audrey had a strong character, but she would never have dared throw a temper tantrum.

What Jerome and Lillian never taught them was to express their spirituality as Audrey did. Brigitte, Jerome's sister and Audrey's godmother, taught her children many more details of piety. In contrast, Jerome and Lillian proposed a simple spiritual life that was spontaneous and elementary: Mass on Sundays and a short prayer at night without too much ceremony.

On any given night, around bedtime, the children would

start yawning, and everything would indicate that the family prayers were about to be forgotten. Audrey, thoughtful and anxious, would delicately hint, "Oh! We haven't prayed!" and watch how everyone would gradually realize it. This ever-present sense of wanting to make her family better, even to the point of imposing her will on them, was totally genuine in her. Her parents and siblings naturally and joyfully gave in to her: "It's Audrey," they would say.

We have already mentioned how Audrey and her big sister complemented each others' characters.

Aline, tranquil and humble, followed her sister like a perfect companion. She admired her, enjoyed her, and derived security from her. Even her shyness would disappear when Audrey was put in charge of a game. And Audrey adored her sister. Aline calmed her impetuous tendencies, laughed at all her jokes, forgave all her excesses, gave in to her desires, listened to her without end, and accepted her just as she was. Audrey worried about Aline, took care of her, tried to defend her at all costs, gave her a place, and made her flourish and shine. She shared her friends and games with her, thanked her infinitely for her patience and humility, and felt responsible for her. At the same time, she found support in Aline and knew she could count on her as a marvelous moderator for her explosive character. Neither one ever put the other down. Their mutual admiration made the two of them a melody of union, gratitude, and mutual praise.

With Henry, it was quite a different story. He was the first boy, and Audrey was two years older than him. He had blond, curly hair. Mummy was very busy with him when he was little, always bringing him along with her and never forgetting his toys. So the girls ended up spending most of their time together, and in the summer they had cousins to play with who were around their age. Audrey was not too pleased with her little brother's monopoly on Mummy's attention. At age three, the little boy's personality began to emerge, and as he grew, he became a stupendous boy, extremely sensible and rather "chic." Yes, Henry was a real dandy. He loved to go out dressed well, with his hair combed just so—parted perfectly on the side. He didn't even get dirty when he played. But he was also filled with the natural vitality of little boys, and he was turbulent and noisy. Aline was always getting him off the hook and making excuses for him when something went wrong.

By contrast, Audrey was strong, serious, ordered, highly reflective, and a master organizer. She would get annoyed with her brother because she couldn't understand his childish anarchy.

"Hey, you took my notebook!" "You ruined my puzzle!" "You're chewing on my pencil!" "And my room…it was all tidy!"

Audrey loved to paint, and she would do so with great concentration. But then Henry would invade her room, imitating an airplane in the process of crashing and suddenly…boom! He would fall on top of her without warning. The peacefulness of the house was in danger. Lillian had two house rules that were absolutely unbreakable: there was to be no bad language and no fighting between brothers and sisters. Never. So she felt that this was serious and that an end had to be put to this problem between Audrey and the vivacious little boy. This time Papa spoke to Audrey. It was the first time Jerome used his paternal authority with Audrey. It was very brief. He took her aside and reminded her, very tenderly but with deep conviction, that Christians don't behave like this. Henry, like every child, was a gift from God and was to be treated as such.

Audrey listened, serious, silent, and very impressed. She said nothing.

A little while later, Lillian had a strange feeling: the silence in the house was not at all normal. She went looking for the children. "Henry! Henry!" She found him in Audrey's room. What a surprise! They were sitting on the floor together; Audrey had invited Henry to play in her room with one of her games. Lillian noted the happy expression on the little boy's face. He had no idea of the act of love and fidelity towards Jesus that his sister was making. This was only the beginning of a beautiful relationship that would lead them to overcome their natural differences and learn to love each other with great affection.

Grégoire was born when Audrey was four. Audrey always had a great predilection for him; it was one of those natural preferences that didn't stem from any apparent reason. One morning, while Lillian was still pregnant with Grégoire, everyone was chatting gaily about what would be the best name for the baby. From bedroom to bedroom, while they folded clothes, made beds, and put away toys, they talked about whether it would be a girl or a boy. At one point, Audrey came out of her room into the hallway and interrupted the ongoing speculation with a firm and definitive affirmation: "It will be a boy, and his name will be Grégoire."

That put an end to the conversation, and nobody dared to raise any doubts about the question ever again. From that very moment, Lillian felt a peaceful certainty that the baby would be a boy.

It was a boy, and they named him Grégoire. Everyone was proud of the fact that Audrey had chosen the name. This gave her certain rights. Grégoire was a charming baby, blond as an angel, but very lively...*very*. For Audrey, he was the "apple of her eye." He was her doll, the one upon whom she developed her maternal instinct for the first time. She cared for him, carried him in her arms, dressed him, and would often issue statements in a very decisive, firm way about what one ought and ought not to do with the baby.

Twenty months later came Beatrice. When Audrey was six, she caught pneumonia, but Beatrice was still just a baby, and Mummy had to spend a lot of time on the littlest ones. So this time, it was Papa who took care of Audrey while she was ill. Even then, Audrey was solicitous and caring, like a real big sister.

"Mummy, go ahead and take a walk in the park with the babies. It doesn't matter if I stay home alone."

She behaved very well during her sickness. Never did she complain. It almost seemed like she didn't need anything or anyone. She spent hours and hours by herself, without company. She thought, sang, played, read, and prayed…. She wasn't able to see her siblings very much because of the possibility of infecting them, but she kept track of them from a distance, letting herself be soothed by the song of a busy household, composed of the noises little children make.

During Audrey's illness, Lillian observed her daughter, had intuitions, and stored them in her heart. She began to wonder: *Bernadette of Lourdes, St. Thérèse of Lisieux…they were sick when they were young. God prepared those chosen souls for a great mission by sending them a sickness early on. And what if Audrey….* Lillian began to feel certain that there was a special spiritual destiny in store for her daughter. She spoke about this with Jerome, and they mentioned it to Father Pierre. They were convinced that this idea was possible and yet, at the same time, they were aware that it was madness to even think of it. This premonition was so strong that Lillian caught herself more than once seized by tears, begging the Lord to spare her daughter.

favorite friends

There were two people that Audrey gave herself to with all her heart: Omer and Hector.

Omer and Caroline, the parents of four girls, had been close friends of Jerome and Lillian's for many years. When Omer first saw Audrey, everyone knew that he and Audrey were meant for each other. Jerome, with a legitimate jealousy, remembers that when Omer was around, he ceased to exist for his daughter. When the two of them met, there was an instant spark of pleasure and joy. Who knows if it hit Omer more than Audrey? No other friend or family member was capable of initiating a relationship with Audrey of such affinity, a relationship in which their mutual understanding became so mysteriously perfect. It was beautiful to see them together.

What did Omer do to fascinate Audrey so much? Omer was not a man of many words. When he visited the family, he just went with the flow, with Audrey in her pirouettes and games, letting her sit on his knees or at his side for as long as she wanted.

He noticed this affection on Audrey's part, but didn't give it too much importance. He accepted it; that was all. They certainly went well together. One's immediate impression of Omer was one of gentleness and realism, of purity and perspicacity, of simplicity and enthusiasm for life. Omer's gaze was very lively, youthful, and clear. He smiled with kindness and had a peaceable and playful way about him. He gave the impression of being bored with the monotony of the adults, with their opinions, critiques, and uncertainties. When this happened, he would move elsewhere: he would fix his attention on a broken bicycle, on a tape recorder that didn't work, or on the lawnmower. This was much more interesting—as interesting as helping Audrey feed her doll.

Her other beloved friend was Hector. He had consecrated his whole life to Jesus Christ. For a certain period of time, Jerome and Lillian had him over frequently, because he accompanied Father Pierre. It appears that Audrey perceived that he had a very sweet soul and a great capacity for wonder. He was a true soul mate. He had a serene and shy respect for beautiful and holy things; he was serious and responsible; he was simple, joyful, and peaceful. Surely he and Audrey shared a common attraction to beauty, and when Hector came over, Audrey would get all excited and enthusiastic. Hector was very much her friend; between the two of them, there was an echo of the words of the Little Prince to the fox: "I know a flower...I think she must have tamed me." Maybe it was because Hector knew how to navigate in Audrey's orbit and be there with her, contemplating, sharing, and being thankful.

Audrey loved to hold on to his arms and stand on top of his feet. They would walk around the entrance hall of the apartment like that, in unison. Hector would have to tell her, "Ok, Audrey. That's enough; I'm getting tired."

In the living room with the others, Audrey would want to continue playing. She would lean over the back of the sofa and do a somersault into the cushion, where Hector would catch her and tenderly straighten her out. What a joy! But all this merrymaking was highly attractive to Henry. He immediately began to imitate his sister, without waiting for her to get off the couch. As one might imagine, the game ended in tears—especially when Audrey got an accidental kick in the head from her brother.

The day of her first Communion in Lourdes, Audrey's eyes were everywhere. She was so small and so eager to see everything. Hector lifted her up onto his shoulders, as on a throne, and there she spent the whole day. He didn't leave her for a second. In the basilica, in the gardens and avenues, in the streets, they walked together. Meanwhile, the people looked on and smiled— "There goes a little queen who's making her first Communion." She lacked nothing. She had Jesus, her crown of flowers, and her good friend.

They often invited Hector to be with them during their family prayer. Audrey took him by the hand and dragged him into the entrance hall. After a Hail Mary led by Hector came the prayer to "Our Lady of the Priesthood." After Aline, Hector also said his petition. Audrey was happy because in this friendship, she shared the deepest dimension: the prayer of a soul that has found Christ as his best Friend.

She also had a little friend her own age: Pierre. They spent hours together, playing and talking peacefully. He was a little boy in Audrey's class, the one she had chosen because he didn't say swear words. Very soon, Pierre began to come to the house to participate in the prayer group initiated by Father Thévenin, "Five Loaves and Two Fishes." Aline knew that when Pierre came to the house, it was exclusively to play with Audrey. That was how it was, and it couldn't be any other way. Resigned, Aline accepted not being with them, but she still wondered what they talked about together. Pierre was a very intelligent and tranquil boy. He was quiet and he listened—he listened to Audrey as she proceeded to set forth her world of certainties, opinions, and convictions about all sorts of things. The other children at school, Papa, the Blessed Mother, Rome, the Legionaries, her artistic future in the circus, what she saw in the street, and what was not at all elegant....

Audrey not only had a perfect harmony with these souls she knew so well, but sometimes she also had an instantaneous surprise attraction to people, which was no less certain for being so sudden. It was intense, a true explosion of friendship and tenderness. This was exactly what happened at the Family Congress in September of 1986. On the last day, Mother Teresa of Calcutta was set to be the keynote speaker. There was great expectation in the large auditorium. It was the climax of a big event to which other important speakers had already contributed: Professor Jerome Lejeune, Mercedes Wilson, the Billings couple, Victor Frankl, etc. After the tiny but great nun of Calcutta had spoken, a small group of children waiting offstage—the children of the organizers of the event—were to come out onto the stage and give a bouquet of flowers to Mother Teresa.

Oh, but the auditorium was so enormous, the lights so blinding, and the applause of so many people.... The children were intimidated and didn't dare to come forward. The organizers encouraged them, "Let's go, let's go. Quickly!" Some seconds went by and nothing happened. Suddenly, when it was least expected, a little blond girl, only three years old, dashed out and threw herself towards Mother Teresa to embrace her. She was so short, so small! It was Audrey. The immense assembly of more than 5,000 participants all rose from their seats and burst into applause, in the midst of laughter and acclamation.

Then there was that occasion at the seminary on Via Aurelia in Rome. It was the first time the family had spent Christmas in Rome, and the Legionaries of Christ had invited them to visit the seminary. God alone knows what kind of fascination those hundreds of smiling young men in their black cassocks exerted upon Audrey. From the seminary, everybody went to St. Peter's Square. Audrey decided to get on the bus with the Legionaries. Aline never even considered it; she ran for the car with Papa and Mummy. Finding it a bit strange, and anxious not to lose sight of her in such a huge crowd, Lillian asked Audrey, "Are you sure you don't want to come with us?" Oh, no. It was too much fun, and there was no way she was getting off the bus. And so, that old Mercedes bus crossed the streets of Rome filled with Legionaries and a little four-year-old girl happily sitting on their knees.

It must have been in one of those jovial moments together when Audrey asked Father Ignacio, LC if he would baptize her doll. And of course, with great pleasure, Father "baptized" it and put it in Audrey's hands. She, in turn, was happy to receive her doll again, since it was *quite* obliged to behave very well from now on.

The Treasure of My Heart

Jerome and Lillian were gradually beginning to understand that Audrey was shielding herself and trying to separate herself from the world. In the beginning, this created problems within the family and with her friends and teachers at school. She didn't mix with the other children when they did things she considered "un-elegant." Jerome and Lillian's adult friends questioned them, asking, "Why do you let this girl close herself off and isolate herself? It only fosters her introversion."

Jerome always held that Audrey was not walling herself off; rather, she was protecting herself. When she refused to attend birthday parties, they asked Father Pierre what to do. Father advised them not to force her, for behind those negative instincts, she was protecting her vocation. At the same time, Jerome was learning—with no small wonder—about the sense of modesty that Audrey had even at a young age. If they went by an indecent advertisement while they were out on the street, she looked away. She didn't watch the scenes on television that were superficial or indecent. Her father tried to figure out where these precocious and spontaneous reactions came from, because the rest of the children normally didn't act the same way.

For the same reasons, Audrey kept a discreet distance from people. For example, when they all arrived at their grandparents' house, Audrey didn't go running to throw herself into their arms as her brothers and sisters did. She wasn't too fond of hugs and kisses; in this area, she was rather austere. She waited at a distance and reflected. Sometimes this attitude bothered others, above all when they were tender and effusive in their affections. It seemed as if she was examining them.

It wasn't pride that made her selective in the area of her affections; rather, it was an instinct of spiritual conservation. Her godmother Brigitte loved her very much. One day, she gave Audrey a necklace and a card with some words which were very much from the heart. Brigitte read Audrey the card and was moved to tears, but she observed how Audrey was disturbed, a bit uncomfortable. Her goddaughter had retreated. She carried a treasure in a vessel of clay; only those who contemplate it are able to understand this behavior.

Her parents received this grace. They knew that all this behavior came from a living, yet mysterious experience. Intuitively, they knew that her eyes were focused on an interior Teacher who educated her, instructed her, and guided her, and they knew that she was always accompanied by him. In the beginning, it was painful for them as parents; nobody wants their child to be educated by "someone else." But before long, they became aware that they were walking on holy ground, and in their souls, they took off their shoes. Audrey and Jesus were friends; Jesus had chosen her as his companion. He wanted to fill her heart with all the delights of his love, and he was initiating a relationship of absolute intimacy with her. He showed how his love is a gratuitous miracle, given with total freedom by pouring his greatness into the heart of a little girl who was perhaps incapable of understanding, of grasping the Mystery, but who was capable of responding to him with total self-giving. Audrey had been invited into the garden of the Beloved. Her soul, the soul of a child and of a woman, hid itself in the cleft of the rock and rested there. There she drank from the wound in the side of her Beloved, and from there, she received her redemptive vocation.

CHAPTER 3

THE TRIAL BEGINS

"My life is nothing more than an instant, a passing hour. My life is nothing more than a single day that escapes me and flees. You know, oh my Lord, that I have only today to love you."

ST. THÉRÈSE OF LISIEUX

A phone call

La Celle St. Cloud. It was August 8, 1990. The phone rang, and Jerome answered. It was Lillian.

"It's happened." Lillian was referring to a conversation she had had with her husband a few months earlier. She had shared with him her fears that Audrey would become seriously ill or have to endure some great suffering. They both had the eerie feeling that "something" was going to happen.

"What is it?"

"Leukemia."

For three days now, they had been a little worried about Audrey's health. They were spending their vacation at Maillot, as they did every summer. "She doesn't feel well. Do you really think it's serious enough to bring her in for a blood test?" Lillian asked Jerome's brother Marc, a doctor in Bordeaux. "She hasn't complained about anything." Upon his advice, Lillian took Audrey to the local doctor for a test.

The next morning at 8:00, the phone rang. The whole family was gathered for breakfast. The doctor wanted Lillian to bring Audrey to his office immediately.

She drove right over with her daughter. With a serious expression on his face, he handed her a sealed envelope and said, "Go right now to the hospital at Caen. Give them this straightaway."

Lillian's heart skipped a beat. She was totally unprepared for that kind of news. The hospital? She was alone. Jerome had gone to Paris. She couldn't let herself cry, and she couldn't bring herself to say anything to Audrey. How different it was to look at her now than it was just a few moments ago. Everything was so terrible and new. Her mind was crowded with questions, with panic. She could already see the faces of her parents, her children, her in-laws, and her friends. Who could help them? And then there was that sense of pressure that weighed on her and took her breath away. Her heart ached. But she knew she had to arm herself with courage.

That same day, she gave the news to the whole family. Jerome called Father Pierre, who was in Lourdes with some families, including Omer and Caroline. Father told them the news right away. They still remember the exact place at the Vert Couret farm where they answered the phone. They went down to the grotto, and everyone put Audrey in Our Lady's hands. Brigitte and Marc were together on a retreat at Paray le Monial, home of Saint Margaret Marie Alacoque. It so happened that the day before the news reached them, Brigitte knelt down to pray in the church, while various people put their hands on her shoulder as they read passages from the Gospel. The priest who was present said in a gentle voice, "I see a great cross over your family that will be a source of many graces." Upon remembering the priest's words the next day, Brigitte was deeply shaken.

In the hospital room at Caen, Lillian cried. She tried to hide it so Audrey wouldn't see.

"What's wrong, Mummy? Do you have allergies in your eyes?"

In any case, at the beginning the doctors thought it was not a very bad case of leukemia. They encouraged them, saying that 80 percent of the patients got well. She could live at home and come once a week to the hospital for ambulatory care, chemotherapy, and blood transfusions.

The symptoms

Audrey was pale and seemed tired, especially during the two weeks before the diagnosis. She had never let on that she felt bad, but she certainly wasn't running around the garden as she used to. The other children jumped and shouted as they always did, but she sat quietly on the steps, just watching. Amazingly, she didn't want to go in the swimming pool. Her clear laughter, like a bell or a rippling stream, was heard less often, but since she didn't complain, nobody suspected that anything serious was amiss. They thought it was just a phase she was going through.

One day, Audrey's paternal grandparents came to visit. They were alarmed upon seeing her. That pallor.... It had been some time since they had seen her, and they noticed a considerable change. Mami suspected it was anemia. That was when Lillian decided to call Marc, Jerome's twin brother and a doctor.

"Take her in for a blood test, and we'll see what it is."

Some weeks after they heard the diagnosis and began the treatment, Lillian asked Audrey, "Are you sure that you were only feeling tired?" Audrey admitted that for over three weeks her bones, arms, and shoulders had been aching.

From that moment on, Audrey's understanding of herself and of her life changed completely. From morning to night, she found herself in front of a steep climb, a painful, uncertain ascent. She had to climb it; there was no way out. The most important hour of her entire life had arrived.

Two days after her entry into the hospital at Caen, Father Thévenin, alerted by Odile, went to visit her. He could read in her soul that Audrey was engaged in combat. They played a game of checkers together, and Father Thévenin watched her closely, gauging her reaction to the various moves. His powerful eyes, the eyes of a friend, of a Father, of an educator, followed her closely. She struggled to win with her child's intelligence. "How can I beat Father Thévenin?" He won. Sitting back in his chair, he looked at her and said:

"Audrey, this is a battle. You have to fight. You have to fight against three armies: your body, your mind, and your spirit. You have to win."

He was wise to speak that way to a sick person. It is the sick person who has to make the decision to live, who has to accept the challenge. Audrey accepted: not just her soul, not just her mind, not just her body, but her entire being took on the challenge.

Some years before, Father Thévenin told the children the secrets of his priestly vocation. In Lisieux, a woman who couldn't
have children asked the bishop if she could spiritually adopt a
seminarian. They assigned her a seminarian named Bruno. Years
later, Father Thévenin, already a parish priest, asked a woman
to help him with some work in the parish. One day, this woman
asked him if there had been two Brunos in the seminary.

"No, just me."

The woman's eyes filled with tears. This was her adopted son,
her seminarian for whom she had so long prayed and sacrificed,
certain that she was keeping watch over his vocation. In those
years, near the end of the seventies, there was a crisis among
some of the French clergy, but he was able to persevere thanks to
that good woman. He was therefore convinced of the urgency to
spiritually adopt priestly vocations in order to guard their vocation. And he was convinced of the power of children's prayers.

Audrey, so tiny and small, understood very clearly what the
priest was telling her. She did not know what was to come or
the mission that would gradually become hers. With childlike
simplicity, she accepted her illness and all that it entailed. She
trusted. Day after day, she let the Lord, *her* Lord, as she affectionately called him, guide her. She was to follow an interior light, a
personal call from Jesus, an invitation: she would offer herself;
she would pray for the conversion of sinners and for vocations,
especially priestly vocations.

TO LIVE THE PRESENT MOMENT

How difficult it must be for a mother to explain to her seven-
year-old daughter that she has leukemia. Lillian didn't know anything about the illness, the treatment, or the course of coming
events. She didn't want to frighten Audrey; she couldn't bear to
make her sad, yet she had always told her children the truth.

Today was no exception. Lillian was also wondering how to say it so that Audrey would be able to live it all in faith. Who is able to teach another to offer her suffering to God?

When Father Thévenin visited Audrey in the hospital, Lillian asked him what to do, and they decided to "let the Lord work in her." But still, she felt that she had to tell her something.

"Audrey, your sickness is serious. I don't know how long you will have to stay in the hospital. We are going to do everything the doctors say."

Audrey's eyes turned to the sky outside the window.

"Mummy, what we are going to do is what Jesus says in the Gospel. We will be like the birds of the sky. We are going to live one day at a time."[1]

Lillian didn't have time to be surprised by this response. In those moments, she came to realize that she didn't know which of them needed more strength. So she let herself be guided by her daughter. Audrey was right: for humble souls, "each day has enough trouble of its own."

From that day on, mother and daughter used this wise advice at every moment. On some occasions, it was impossible not to be worried, not just for today without thinking of tomorrow, but also for the next five minutes: painful, atrocious, extreme minutes. Then the two of them, draining the cup of the present moment, repeated their prayer: "Help me. My Lord, give me strength. I trust in you."

In other circumstances, when Lillian was worrying about something small:

"Dear, I don't know if I will be able to come tomorrow. I have to go buy shoes for Grégoire and Beatrice."

Audrey would respond: "Mummy, don't worry. We'll see each other tomorrow."

---

1. Matthew 6:26-34

That Gospel attitude was the source of serenity for Audrey and her mother during her entire sickness. There, Lillian found the light and strength to sustain her daughter in the hours of agony that followed a session of chemotherapy. There, she found the strength to end the day with faith and love, and to keep from rebelling when she relived it all on the way home from the hospital.

None of those who accompanied Audrey in her sickness saw her worried even for an instant. Her calm expression and her peace were never broken. Those surrounding her struggled with their own worries, battles, and desperation, but she had reached her own conclusion just after her arrival at the hospital in Caen.

"Mummy, I already know why God has sent me this sickness. I believe that he wants to remind me that I must be a good Carmelite."

Audrey did not worry. She did not ask even a single question: *What are they going to do to me? When will I come out of the hospital? Will I be home for Christmas? What will happen if...?* She kept silent. One word: Here I am, Lord. Present. In silence, present. With a prayer, present. With a smile, present. In gratitude and in pain, in the hour of battle and in times of strength...present.

The children in my room at Caen

In the hospital in Caen, Audrey shared a room with other children. Their mothers and relatives came to visit them—country people with Normandy accents and simple manners who filled the room with their humorous conversation. Audrey listened with curiosity and enjoyment, making friends day by day, until the mother of one of the children happened to mention that she had three children, none of whom were baptized. One morning, Lillian found Audrey radiant with joy.

"Mummy, guess what? The lady told me that she has decided to baptize her three children!"

"Oh, that's wonderful!" replied Lillian. Nevertheless, she didn't give this too much importance because she was more concerned about how Audrey was doing. They were waiting for the doctors to tell them whether Audrey could spend the weekend at home. Finally, they got the yes. What excitement, what joy! To have a child in the hospital was such a trial for the family, so it was a great joy for everyone to have her home again.

Everyone came by to see her in her room, in the garden, in the dining room. Of course, she couldn't go swimming in the pool, even though it was hot outside. She couldn't run, and they had to keep a strict watch over her diet. But on Sunday they were able to go to Mass as a family, with Audrey and Granny hand-in-hand. The parish priest knew his parishioners well, and he knew the locals from the vacationers. He had been told that Audrey was sick. After Mass was over, he came out, as usual, under the portico, where people greeted each other, laughed together, chatted, asked for advice, and invited each other for a drink or a cup of coffee. This time, the priest went directly to Audrey's family. After giving the other children a friendly pat, he bent down to greet Audrey.

The priest asked her endless questions and made numerous observations about her appearance, her health, the first days in the hospital, her family. It looked like Audrey wanted to say something, but the priest never stopped talking. Audrey bit her lips and looked anxiously at her mother. She wanted to speak. She looked back at the priest, impatiently waiting her chance. Because of her good manners, she did not interrupt; she kept still and waited. When she could, she slipped a word in edgewise:

"Father, may I ask you something?"

"Yes, my dear child. What is it?"

"I would like you to pray today for three children who are going to be baptized. They are three brothers, and one was with me in the hospital. Please, don't forget to pray very much for them!"

"Yes, of course, for the children. Ah, they will be baptized, eh?

Yes, that's very important, very important. I will pray for them!" promised the priest, glancing at Lillian with surprise. He was not able to understand why a little girl from Paris who was sick with leukemia should be so interested in some country children who were going to be baptized.

This was another of Audrey's defining traits during her sickness. If she was selfless before her sickness, always thinking of the needs of others, now she was almost unable to think of herself. Her sensitivity to others had grown to such a degree that she had completely stopped thinking of herself.

The graces she undoubtedly received through her suffering with leukemia were transforming those divine seeds that had been stored up like a growing treasure since the tender years of her childhood, and now they were ready to burst into full bloom. Generosity, prayer, and sacrifice offered always for others…her heart was reaching a keen understanding that the crucified Jesus had come to save what was lost.

At Home Again

Towards the end of August, the family settled once again in the house on Jules Verne Street, in La Celle St. Cloud, near Versailles.

During the back-to-school season, the Lafayette and Printemps department stores were full of mothers and children. The cashiers rang up notebooks, pencils, Hello Kitty stickers. In Paris, the Metro and the advertisements showed a little blond boy with a photogenic smile, wearing a sweater and a scarf, and sporting a brightly colored knapsack. In front of the school, the parents stood in a long line during roll call, waiting for their child's name to be read out and his classroom assigned. Lillian waited her turn, her mind and gaze elsewhere. Since the girls had entered their new school only last April, she didn't know the other mothers very well.

"How are you, Madame? It's for the fourth and fifth grades, right? Your daughters are called…Aline and Audrey."

"No, it's just Aline."

"Oh, yes?"

"Yes. Audrey is home sick. It's leukemia."

"Oh my! What did you say, Madame? A daughter with leukemia? That's terrible!"

The news raced around the school like wildfire. The ladies talked about it together.

"And who is this girl?"

"Audrey, it's Audrey."

"Oh, her poor parents."

"But I don't remember her very well. Oh, of course—they came in April."

"Yes, in April."

A little seven-year-old girl said, "Mummy, I know who Audrey is. She's the new girl who gave away her snack every day. She gave me some a few times."

During September, Lillian was bringing Audrey to the hospital for blood transfusions and chemotherapy twice a week. This was the first stage of the treatment. Nevertheless, they still didn't know exactly what kind of leukemia was attacking her system, and they were hoping that she would begin to respond between the fourth and sixth weeks of chemotherapy. At the moment, they didn't know if the prognosis was good, but they did know it wasn't all bad.

Aline came home from school, feeling at a loss without her sister. She didn't understand her math homework, and school was weighing on her. "Audrey doesn't have to go to school—she's free of all that! No, but she's sick. What's going to happen to her?" She felt happy coming home because Audrey was there. Oh, but now there was a lady with her. Who was that?

"How are you, Aline? I'd like you to meet Mrs. Barbé. She has come to give me classes and she will come every day. That way, I won't fall behind in school."

The teacher was not very young, but she had a friendly air about her. She smiled a lot and explained everything as if it were a story. With her, grammar, numbers, and historical characters all danced, moved, and seemed to come alive. Audrey watched her speak: her luminous eyes, her red hair, her curls, her expressive hands full of freckles....

Mrs. Barbé had been dedicated to teaching and entertaining sick children in hospitals and at their homes for quite some time. She had the sweetest gaze, and there was no question that she and Audrey got along well from the start. Audrey, insatiable, wanted to do everything fast, and so they went from one activity to the next.

"Let's go over the verbs, and then you can give me a dictation. Will that leave us enough time to do mathematics? But before you leave, we have to practice some acting, like in the theater."

Audrey had one worry: she didn't want to fall behind in school if she could help it. Mrs. Barbé perceived this, and although she knew it wasn't possible, she didn't want to shatter Audrey's hopes.

Aline was trying to finish her work at the dining room table, and she kept looking over at them. It was obvious that she couldn't concentrate, and she was having a hard time. Audrey and Mrs. Barbé were having so much fun! Audrey's gaze followed her sister.

"Mrs. Barbé, could you help my sister a little with her homework?"

The shadow of the cross

Audrey's new hospital was called Robert Debré, and it was located on the eastern edge of Paris. It was a huge hospital, the most modern in the city, exclusively for children. Her first contact with that new world left certain impressions. All of the hospital staff were mysteriously adorned, neatly dressed in white and green. Audrey observed the doctors and the nurses and noticed their different uniforms. She wanted to know everything.

"Why does that doctor wear all green with a kind of cover on his shoes? And what is that little cap?"

"He is a surgeon, and that's how they dress for operations."

"And why does this nurse wear white pants while the others wear skirts and stockings?"

In a little while, she would come to know each member of this new family, and not only by their uniforms. There was a whole discipline, a distinctive way of dealing with people, and a diversity of categories to take into account. There were the night-shift nurses, the women who brought food to the patients, the cleaning staff, the nurses aides who came to bathe the patients and change the sheets, and the doctors who kept watch over the patients. And then there was the professor, who was the most important doctor, responsible for a whole section of the hospital, along with his two assistants, who were also very important.

The nurses examined Audrey without saying a single word, with their face masks in place. She couldn't see them very well, and she had to remain almost naked, wearing only her underpants. She didn't like this strange new sensation. People passed by in the corridor, some in wheelchairs and some in stretchers. It really began to seem like she was sick. Her eyes traveled everywhere; she gazed deeply at the rest of the patients. She was a bit frightened to see a group of doctors and nurses who were running with a stretcher. One was holding the oxygen, the other the serum, while the boy on the stretcher looked pale, his eyes closed. Poor boy. A chill ran up Audrey's spine; the pure novelty of it all gave her the shivers. Mummy couldn't enter all of the examining rooms with her, and all of those faces were so unfamiliar. Later on, she would become an expert, perfectly familiarized and used to everything.

"Lay back and don't breathe. Okay, now you can breathe."

She would get to know all of those electronic devices with numbers in red, yellow, and green, the modern consoles full of buttons, and the beeps and noises when all the equipment started up. But now it frightened her when the lights suddenly changed from incandescent to darkness.

For Lillian, too, all of this was a new world. She would never forget the first chemotherapy session. She slept fitfully and had to get up early to drive Audrey to the hospital, which was quite a distance away from the house. As soon as the alarm clock went off, she leapt out of bed and lunged towards the door of her room. Opening it with a nervous jerk, she found Audrey standing there, perfectly serene, quiet, immaculately dressed and combed.

"Good morning, Mummy."

Audrey spent her first night in the hospital, and Mummy went to see her in the morning. She found her peaceful and in good spirits. They spent some time together talking and looking at each other. But Audrey had to get up every few minutes to go into the bathroom. After an hour, Lillian asked, "Audrey, why are you so restless?"

"It's because I'm throwing up."

It turned out that she had spent the whole night vomiting. She hadn't called the nurse; she hadn't said anything. Lillian was horrified.

"Audrey, why didn't you say anything? You have to tell us so that we can take care of you better."

In those first days, Audrey continued to avoid showing signs of discomfort or pain. Mummy became tense. Audrey hid her discomfort and endured in silence. She resisted. Then, Mummy had to become firmer with her:

"Audrey, you have to tell us what is going on, even though you don't want to. These doctors want to cure you. We all want you to get better, but we need you to help us. You have to tell us what hurts."

It was very difficult to convince her. But finally, from then on, she would occasionally admit that she had a "little bit of pain." She didn't complain, either about the pain or about being forced to speak against her will.

A Gift for Jesus

A cold, gray November 9th. Mummy and Papa weren't at home. Grégoire and Beatrice were happily occupied with the young nanny; Henry went here and there, and Aline studied verbs for the next day. Audrey had been in the hospital for a few days. She was tired, very tired.

Lillian found out the news late in the day. She went straight from the hospital to her in-laws' house to get Jerome, who was having dinner there. The professor's assistant had told her that Audrey had not responded to the chemotherapy. The results of the cario-type were not good. She had been diagnosed with acute lymphoblastic leukemia, of which there are several kinds. Normally, these patients responded positively to the treatment by the fourth or sixth week of chemotherapy. However, the latest results of the tests had revealed that the prognosis was wrong because there had been an error in the diagnosis. Audrey's type of leukemia was "Pre B," which indicated a grave chromosomal deformation; her DNA was damaged. And how does one heal that? It required a bone marrow transplant with a very small probability of success.

They began a series of extremely strong chemotherapy sessions. Lillian, in her gentle, tender way, had explained to Audrey that the treatment would cause her to lose all of her hair. She knew how much her daughter loved her hair, since she considered it the only pretty feature she had. After a little while, she said, "Mummy, I believe I will be the first nun in France to offer her hair to Jesus twice."

When one enters the Carmelite Order, one's hair is cut off; Audrey had decided she would accept the sacrifice with joy. This circumstance was unexpected, yet she had taken to the idea, and she offered it with the same joy.

Seeing that Audrey was losing her beautiful, long, blond hair was very painful to her mother. But she became really alarmed when she realized that her little girl was also losing her eyebrows and eyelashes. She confided her horror to Granny who wisely replied: "She will always keep her *regard.*" Yes, Lillian thought, Audrey's *regard:* that expression in her eyes, so penetrating, yet so gentle. Her gaze when she looked at her picture of Jesus. Her loving gaze when she looked at Aline. Her bright look as Mummy came into the room. The look that reflected her soft smile.

The Tuesday Rosary

Every morning, Jerome went to Les Châtaigniers school to drop off Aline and Henry. His blond head stood out in the entrance of the school among the crowd of mothers. He gave a kiss to each of them, adjusted their scarves, and off they went. With his hands in his pockets, he watched them run off and mingle with the rest of the children. How cold it was outside! Some of the ladies asked him about Audrey, and he explained the relapse. Cold outside; cold inside—and tears. One of the ladies exclaimed, "We have to do something! Listen, everyone come next Tuesday to my house. We'll offer a Rosary together for Audrey." The idea was passed on by word of mouth.

On Tuesday at 8:15 p.m., Jerome, Aline, and Henry arrived at the appointment and were met with a surprise. So many children! There were almost twenty of them, all between the ages of six and eleven. About ten families had come. The hosts opened up their living room, pushed back the sofas, brought chairs from the dining room, and got everyone settled. All of them took their places in front of an image of Our Lady that had previously been kept in storage. One woman kept count on an antique rosary; it had been years since it had been taken out of its keepsake box. A boy was showing off the rosary he had gotten for his first holy Communion, which he had just made last May. The Hail Marys flowed. Most people counted on their fingers. There was a mistake from time to time because people were out of the habit. The eyes of the adults softened as they listened to each others' voices—the voices of the men and of the women.

Jerome's voice was strong. He had never prayed the Rosary in public before. Everyone was asking Mary for the healing of an innocent and generous little girl. Without realizing it, and in an instinctive, deep, and vital way, they were begging for the healing of their own sicknesses: the most hidden wounds, the most secret pains, the unconfessed wrongdoings. There was a very special atmosphere in the making here; before Mary, all of them were defenseless children. The prayer for "her" was changed into a prayer for "us." They ended with a little song.

The most determined children, their spirits lifted by the familiar melody, raised their voices and led the song. Most people hid their voices, choking back their emotion.

In the hospital, Lillian gave Audrey the news: "Did you know? This evening some friends are going to pray a Rosary for you."

Lillian was hesitant to mention how concerned others were about Audrey. These were people Audrey didn't even know. Lillian had no idea how Audrey would react, and she didn't like to tell her about all the interest and spiritual efforts her case had stirred up. As usual, Audrey took the information as a matter of course and responded simply, but with resolve, from the depths of her heart:

"I will pray the Rosary with all of them from the hospital, and I will offer it for each one of them."

Audrey always prayed for others. It had become almost an obsession. And she worried about choosing intentions for her prayers in a very concrete way. She prayed all the time, especially in the moments of pain. In those moments, she and Mummy turned to their intentions. It was as if she feared to lose even a second of her Calvary, as if even that did not belong to her....

Children and adults began to get involved in the Tuesday Rosary. There was a special light in the eyes of everyone, a shared desire. They decided to get together every Tuesday, each time in a different house. The children rejoiced at the news: it would mean, among other things, going to bed a little later that night—what fun! And so it was that the Tuesday Rosary became a custom. Different people came every week as the invitation was spread by word of mouth. Even Jerome missed it on several occasions; he did so in order to show that there was no obligation to come every week. Those who came were those who had a real desire to pray. As the weeks went by, the number of people increased. Some children even came in their pajamas. An older couple came from the same neighborhood of Versailles. Little by little, the rosary group was taking shape. As it grew in numbers, Jerome took to handing around a little basket with rosaries of all kinds. The fingers of the children eagerly dug through the basket. "The yellow one for me!" "I want the one with the wooden beads!"

The children always led the fifth mystery, a privilege for which they eagerly waited. They had a special sense that if Audrey were cured, it would be because of their prayers. In each session, they spontaneously chose who would lead each mystery. On one occasion, Jerome was distributing the decades and he noticed a man whom he had never seen before.

"Would you mind leading the third mystery?"

When the moment arrived, the mystery didn't start. Jerome made a signal to the gentleman. His daughter, seated as his feet, began:

"Hail Mary...."

"Hail Mary," repeated her father.

"Full of grace..." continued the girl.

"Full of grace," he followed, looking at his daughter.

That night, a little girl taught her father to pray the Hail Mary.

The Tuesday Rosary had an impact on the people who came, not only a social or religious impact, but a personal one also. There were families that had never gotten together to pray the Rosary, couples that had never prayed together, homes that had never hosted people to pray. One night, one of the ladies said, "I never imagined that so many people would come to my house to pray." For almost two years, this Rosary would be a true psychological and moral support for Lillian, Jerome, and their children. The people who came were nourished by the living example of Audrey, and they grew spiritually. Because of it, many homes began to welcome prayer.

Every Tuesday the children met with Audrey in prayer. Here was a girl their age who was suffering in her hospital bed. How many good resolutions she inspired in her little friends! Among these children, friendships have been formed that time has not been able to erase. In their childhood memories, there is an indelible mark of those Tuesdays, the Virgin Mary, and Audrey.

One Tuesday, a grandmother who was participating in the Rosary could not go. The night before, inspired, she had written a small acrostic[2] about Audrey. She sent it with her family to make herself present among them.

A *mour infinie du Père,*
U *ni a la compassion du Fils, nous te supplions,*
D *élivre Audrey des filets de la maladie.*
R *edonne-lui, par ton Esprit, la santé de l'âme et du corps nous te supplions.*
E *ternelle sera notre louange à*
Y *ahvé, tout puissant, notre Dieu. Amen.*

---

2. Translation: Infinite love of the Father, united to the compassion of the Son, we beg you: deliver Audrey from the snare of sickness. By your Spirit, give her health again in soul and body. Eternal will be our praise to Yahweh all-powerful, our God. Amen.

From that day on, they prayed this prayer every Tuesday at the end of the Rosary. Jerome and Lillian had a photo of Audrey printed with the acrostic prayer on the back. They handed it out to the people they met and asked for their prayers. The mysterious force of love would spread this photograph literally to the ends of the earth. In the most isolated corners of the country, this prayer was recited; it was found in the deepest recesses of the home; it was carried about in purses, agendas, and wallets. Father Thévenin gave it out to all the children of the Theresian mission. Every family in the school had it. It landed in the hands of many Legionaries of Christ.

Jerome sent a package of photographs to Rome, to be given out to bishops and members of the Curia—with the hope that one would reach the hands of the Holy Father. From Rome, the photograph arrived in Japan. During a trip, it fell into the hands of a French seminarian who was working in Tokyo and who had been adopted by Aline through the Theresian mission. Various priests spread it about through monasteries and cloistered convents.

Many nuns in France, hidden between vineyards and mountains or in the heart of a metropolis, knew of Audrey. In Bordeaux, a convent of Poor Clares was suffering from a lack of vocations. They put the photo of Audrey on the altar and entrusted this intention to her.

Brigitte, who lived in Lyon, dedicated herself to spreading the photograph everywhere she went. One day, she was at Mass in the Basilica of Fourrières when a lady came up to her after the ceremony and said, "Excuse me, I would like to give you this photo. It is a young girl who is suffering from leukemia, and we have to pray a great deal for her to get well."

Brigitte's eyes misted over with tears. It was the picture of her goddaughter. It was Audrey.

Last sacraments

Two priests with Roman collars and briefcases went up the elevator to the fifth floor. They walked down the corridor, much to the surprise of the nurses who looked at them with distrust, irony, and wonder. What are these two priests doing in a hospital? In secular France, public hospitals were strictly lay establishments and normally, no one could enter dressed like that. The hospital was "for everyone." Two days earlier, Jerome had asked Father Pierre to give Audrey the sacrament of the sick. Father Hector was at hand, so Father Pierre brought him along.

The room they wanted was the last one on the corridor, the most isolated, across from the sterile bubbles.[3] Upon approaching the door, they could hear cries. Nurses went swiftly in and out of the room. A doctor rushed to the scene and glanced at them quickly on his way into the room. They stepped aside. He entered the room hurriedly and closed the doors. Father Hector and Father Pierre glanced at one another. They were worried. Those cries—what was happening to the girl? Jerome came out pale and frightened. The situation was not normal.

"Nothing happened to her, but she's desperate and in great pain. She's been like this for a quarter of an hour."

Audrey was writhing in pain. Desperation, cries, tears. She was soaked, her closed eyes trying to endure, her hands clenched. She moved and shook.

It was painful for everyone. The doctors could not explain it. Jerome entered the room again, visibly nervous. The priests stayed waiting for half an hour, and then approached the girl.

"Audrey, Audrey, listen. The priests have come to give you

---

3. A "sterile bubble" is a small room that is kept completely sterilized and isolated from the external world. It is used as a protective measure for patients with weakened immune systems.

the sacrament of the sick. Audrey, you have to calm down. They are waiting for you." There was no way. She got even worse. "Audrey, I know that you can't answer me. Don't worry. Just make a little gesture for me. Do you want the priests to give you the sacrament?"

She nodded her head "yes" without being able to stop the tears. She kept her eyes shut. They had Father Pierre enter. That was a challenge. Father prepared himself, putting on the stole, taking up the missal. He began to recite the prayers with a firm voice. His voice was lost in between the cries of the girl, yet he continued. As much as he could, he drew near to Audrey. Father Hector was going to trace the sign of the cross on her forehead with the holy oil. The sheets would get stained. Father would get stained. No matter, it had to be done. He marked her forehead with the holy oil and withdrew his hand.

What happened? Complete calm. Complete silence. Audrey relaxed and recovered her normal breathing. She stopped flinching. Everyone breathed a sigh of relief and yet could not contain their surprise. Two nurses came running with tranquilizing drugs, but they were too late. The pain had passed, had gone away. Jerome drew near to his little daughter, his face next to hers.

"Audrey, truly, today you conquered the devil."

saint Andrew

Not everyone caught Audrey's name the first time they were introduced. Her name was English, uncommon in France. But many people resolved the unfamiliarity by saying, "Ah, yes! *Andrée*," and were quite satisfied with that.

On the 30th of November, the feast day of St. Andrew, Lillian realized what day it was and mentioned it to Audrey:

"Audrey, today is the feast of St. Andrew. Remember all those people who thought your name was Andrew?"

Audrey looked at her mother with a little smile.

"Mummy, I prefer to choose St. Andrew as my patron."

"But why? Saint Audrey has such a beautiful story! She was an Anglo-Saxon princess. She went through a thousand adventures, and she had a great heart and defended her faith up to the point of heroism."

"Yes, I know." A moment of silence. "But Saint Andrew was chosen by Jesus himself and left everything to follow him."

Hospital scenes

Mummy arrived with the video recorder. Yesterday, Audrey had sent Aline a message in code so that only she would understand it. Lillian was filming her every day so that her brothers and sisters would see her, and then afterwards, she would film them at home so that Audrey could keep track of everyone's life more closely. Aline answered her message. The little children appeared in the dining room making faces. Beatrice said, "Hi, Audrey!" Audrey laughed. These were the little joys that crossed her night of pain like a comet. She spent her days with her mother; her brothers and sisters could not come to see her. During these months, only Aline had been given special permission. Audrey sent her letters, some of them in an extremely complicated code that she spent hours making. Each letter of the alphabet corresponded to a little invented drawing, and entire sentences would be assembled out of drawings. Afterwards, Aline would receive the "alphabet" and would comb through it in order to decipher the message.

Jerome now had to take care of the little ones at home, playing both Mummy and Papa. A young nanny helped him, but it was always necessary to tie a shoe, carry a resistant little one to the bathtub, fix the pieces of a game, and just be there. Every day, Papa received a telephone call around five in the afternoon. It was Audrey. Lillian usually left the hospital around 4:00 or 5:00, leaving her alone.

"See you tomorrow, dear. I leave you with *Little House on the Prairie*. When it ends, give me a call."

Audrey half-watched the television, but she was suffering. When Lillian arrived home, she would then call Audrey on the phone. Jerome knew Audrey needed her mother, for it was in her arms that she was navigating this storm. It was so difficult to remain alone. He knew; he was also a little alone. He answered the phone. "How are you, Audrey?"

"Has Mummy arrived?"

"No, not yet."

On the highway, Lillian drove past Clichy, past Asnières, all the way around to the west of Paris, out beyond Saint Cloud, Versailles. The traffic was heavy coming out of Paris, but Lillian moved right along without delay.

The uncertainty of those days.... Her children entrusted to Providence. That mystery of Audrey's prayer. The human faces that passed by in the hospital corridors. White and green scrubs, the smell of disinfectant. Oxygen, serum. *When is this going to end?* A car passes her on the right. Traffic is stopped in the tunnel. Delayed. *Lord, give me strength.* Starting off again. Evening falls.

Jerome and Audrey, united by the phone receiver, wait. For a moment, Audrey's room has the feel of existential emptiness. A sad feeling of desertion envelops her and fills her with fears. Jerome breathes. He is there, at her side.

"Okay, dear. We're going to sing a song."

Lillian puts on her blinker. Exit: Versailles. When she arrives, she finds Audrey and Papa singing. Audrey and Papa crying.

"The Lord has done great things for me, holy is his name."

Through the night, Audrey remains alone. She is in bed, in her place, the center from which she organizes her life. Her control tower...her operations center. She has to fill the loneliness in new ways. Here, she cannot see the reflection of the light filtering through the shutters, the way it did during her naps at Maillot: little balls of sun danced on the wall, now in a line, now separated. Lines of light on the ceiling: now they moved; now they were still. There, you played by watching and watching: the light, the blinds.... Now there were no windows. Now there was no sun. Everything was hermetically sealed. Your gaze slipped from the wall to the ceiling, from the ceiling to the IV tube, from the tube to the night table: pill boxes, disposable handkerchiefs, two pencils, a ripped envelope without its letter.

The hours flowed by like the drops of IV fluid. The noise of the cars grew louder; the highway was getting busy now. Everyone had already had their breakfast, and now they were going to work, to school. For her, it was all the same; all the noises sounded the same. Even the time seemed not to change, except perhaps on those days when there was something different. From far away, far above, she heard the sound of a dog barking. It had been months since she had seen or heard a dog barking.

Her foot wrinkled the sheets; they were the same sheets as yesterday. They would come to change them at nine o'clock, but it was still early. *I wrinkle them, I stretch them, I try to tell whose steps and voices I hear. Now the nurse puts the food on the serving trays. Now she is filling a glass with water. Now she is going into the room next door. She puts everything down and says nothing. The nurses say nothing. Now she goes out. But no, she hasn't gone out! Why hasn't she gone out? I will ask the nurse to tell me a story. Ah, but surely she doesn't know any stories. Granny tells me lots of stories. Yesterday that nurse forgot her magazine on the windowsill. A page was left opened. There was a picture of a naked woman. I didn't want to look at it. What for? Let them take it away. I pull up the covers and turn over in the bed so as not to see it.*

When Aline visits on Sundays with Papa, they don't talk

much. They just play. They always play what Audrey wants, but Audrey always wants whatever Aline wants. Audrey likes to see Aline laughing. Audrey looks at Aline's hair; Audrey no longer has any. She looks at Aline's hands, her clothes. It's Aline.

When Audrey gets tired, she doesn't say so. She suggests a new game. Ah, but no. If I have to take pills, better to keep playing the same game. Lillian sits at her side. Audrey concentrates and tenses up. Aline has never heard her complain. She doesn't realize what is going to happen. Water and little pills of all colors...the bottles have instructions on them, written by hand. Lillian is serious, attentive, rereading the instructions.

"Come on, Audrey, let's take these."

"No, Mummy."

It was a surprise for Aline. Her sister didn't want to take a pill. Lillian insisted. Audrey whimpered and leaned back in bed. It was beginning to become a scene. Aline was amazed, because Audrey did not normally make scenes. Lillian became firm and serious.

"Audrey, you have to."

Finally, the pill approached her lips and was put into her mouth. She spat it out! Aline was shocked. She didn't understand this behavior. It was just a little pill.... Audrey would not be conquered by it. Even in her sickbed, she would not be deprived of one whit of her vitality. But what was going on inside.... Lillian knew a little, but the only one who really knew was Audrey.

Chemotherapy terrified her. Under her shirt, they place a catheter that goes directly into her heart; they connect her to the tubes and program the machine. Fear in the skin. Fear in the eyes. Then it all begins. All the chemicals start to enter in—drugs to attack and kill the cancer and many other things as well. There is general alarm in the organism. It seems like a hostile army is entering into the body and will take no prisoners. The immune system, or what's left of it, prepares itself, badly wounded, for a counterattack. Total exhaustion, extreme discouragement.... And then it is finished.

But now comes the worst of all: carrying the venom inside. Now, to resist. Fatigue, nausea, open cuts on the inside of your mouth, skin so dry that it bleeds...that sensation of powerlessness. The shadow of the cross. The shadow of the nails. Then comes the exhausting vomiting. Everything hurts, even the bones inside, as if someone had put broken shards of glass in them. It's like gout, but in the marrow of the bones. The muscles hurt, the eyes hurt. The fever rises, and you tremble and sweat. It hurts to breathe; it burns inside. The chemicals cause a general inflammation of the internal passageways, which are trying to defend themselves from that interior fire. It burns, irritates, wounds. That is why it is infinitely painful to swallow. It makes you want to scream; it makes you want to cry—but your mouth hurts so much that you can barely open it. It is swollen, wounded, inflamed by the medicine, and attacked for lack of defenses.

Beyond the doors of this agony, there were some very nice and well-dressed ladies who walked from room to room, kind and smiling. They were *Les Dames Roses* (the Pink Ladies) who came to entertain the children. Some days they were told, "Audrey can't play today." But on other days, yes, of course she could. There was the nice lady who taught one how to paint with those pretty pictures of animals. And the one who taught knitting! This interested Audrey very much, although she thought her grandmother did it much better. She gave it a lot of attention and care. If she didn't finish, she asked the lady to come back again the next day. That border couldn't be left like that.

Mami tried to help Lillian however she could. On Wednesdays, she would go to the hospital to review verbs and conjugations with Audrey, leaving her house with everything prepared: the leather purse, the silk scarf, the grammar books. Today, she decided, she would try to get Lillian to come down to the hospital cafeteria to have lunch. Lillian needed to nourish herself and get a change of atmosphere. After lunch was the session of classes with Audrey, whose desire to learn was insatiable. She repeatedly told Mami that she didn't want to repeat a grade and had to keep up to date. It gave her great security to receive her grandmother's approval because she "knows a lot." Partway through the lesson, Mami proposed a game of cards, but Audrey was firm: "No, Mami, we have to finish these three sentences."

Mami arrived back at her house on the avenue de Villiers. She was tired. As she went up in the elevator, she said to herself, *That girl—her strength comes from within, her strength comes from within.*

purity

Audrey's hospital took in children with terminal illnesses, and the staff was trained specifically in the treatment of children. Nevertheless, and contrary to what one might expect, the doctors' and nurses' dealings with the children were cold, distant, and impersonal. A nurse would not tend to the same child more than two or three days in a row. It was a hospital norm. There was a very understandable reason for this: to avoid creating affective bonds between the staff and their patients that could become inconvenient. If the nurse developed too much of an affection for a child and the child died, she could become affected and experience a strong frustration that might lead her to abandon her work. In fact, this had happened more than a few times, and it was no small problem for the hospital administration. To lose nurse after nurse almost overnight for sentimental reasons—and this after a specialized and difficult training.... It was totally forbidden for a doctor or a nurse to establish a friendship with the children and families of the patients. There were many children in the hospital, and each one was a world in itself, full of suffering and drama.

The staff had to do everything possible in order to save them and had to be able to give the same treatment to all of them.

But for the children this was tremendously hard, for in extreme situations they showed a very intense need for affection. A child pulled away from his nest is like a little abandoned bird peeping helplessly in the midst of a storm. They have stripped him of the familiar smells of his own room, his bed, his hallway, his kitchen, the sounds of his brothers and sisters at play, and the continual contact with his mother and father. Here in the hospital, not only did he feel the absence of his own family, but he was treated coldly by that unknown group of people who were taking care of him.

Audrey looked at the nurses with much attention. She tried to meet their averted eyes.

"What's your name?"

Only a little conversation; she waited impatiently for the door to open again. She saw her coming. There were the footsteps, the cart with the IV fluid…but now it was not the same person. What had happened?

"She will come later."

But later never arrived. Audrey had to get used to the system the hard way. It had already happened on a few occasions. Once, when she discovered that a night nurse was Catholic, she stayed awake into the early hours of the morning waiting to greet her and speak with her for a few moments. Later, when she went to Lourdes, she bought a religious medal for her, but they didn't allow her to give it to the nurse in the hospital. The staff was forbidden to receive anything from the children. Something similar happened with a doctor, one of the first who took care of Audrey. Lillian still didn't know the system. The doctor seemed very nice, and she thought they would have a lot of contact with him. Audrey was charmed. The doctor once arrived in her room with a guitar to sing her some songs. It seems that word of this got around, for they never saw him again.

Now they brought Audrey on a stretcher to a room surrounded by big windows and prepared her for some tests. She went alone, without Mummy. A nurse stripped her down completely without saying a single word.

"Stay here lying down and don't move."

Audrey trembled from pure discomfort and from the unpleasantness of it all. Defenseless, she was stripped in front of everyone, and she felt unprotected and humiliated. A man came in with a white dressing gown to cover her. He smiled, gave her a little pat, and left. Then came a doctor and another person, along with the assistant nurses who push the buttons. There were five people around her bed. Around her naked little body, they discussed her case, exchanged opinions, examined her eyes, joked, turned her over, and drew their conclusions. There was a friendly gesture of farewell, and they left. She stayed there, at the mercy of a grotesque and unfamiliar environment. She didn't like these things at all; she had already suffered something similar that time at Maillot.

"We're going to take a picture!"

She was about five years old. Omer's two girls, Aline, and Audrey were put in line, naked in the tub, by height. They were so cute. Oh, but Audrey appeared in the photo with a contrary expression on her face. She didn't like that at all; it was her virginal instinct that led her to preserve herself from the eyes of the world. Maybe that was why she had insisted from the beginning of her stay in the hospital that the male nurses must not bathe her. It was out of the question.

"I only want Mummy to bathe me."

Mummy, Audrey's companion along her path, the sister of her prayer, the confidante of her most intimate secrets: discreet, respectful, deep. Mummy, who contemplated the work of the Lord on her knees, with her shoes off and kneeling, like one who walked on sacred ground.

This morning, she was visited by a young, handsome, and friendly doctor.

"Good morning, my little rabbit."

Audrey stiffened and put herself on guard. When he left the room, the doctor pinched a nurse, giving her a flirtatious look. This was absolutely not elegant. As the days went by, it disgusted Audrey that this doctor came to examine her. Now, she was his "little bunny, his little dove." She was bothered by the giggles of the nurses in the corridor when the doctor came out of the room.

"Mummy, I don't like it when he calls me 'my little rabbit.'"

"Audrey, it's no big deal."

"Well, if he likes animals so much, he should be a veterinarian."

One day it was the last straw. The doctor sat on her bed to examine her. She bristled like a porcupine and looked at him with severity, shrinking back from the doctor's hands. He became displeased.

"That's enough! You're refusing to let yourself be examined, aren't you?"

"Yes," responded Audrey with a strong and dry tone, looking directly into his eyes.

The doctor stood up, took off the smock, and left the room almost shouting, "I'm not going to deal with you anymore—find another doctor!"

He complained about the girl's behavior to his superior. "She's a brat. She doesn't let me examine her; she has something against me."

Lillian spoke with Audrey. "Audrey, why are you so negative with that doctor?"

"I don't like him; I don't like how he behaves with the nurses."

"Yes, Audrey, but understand that he is not Christian. Nobody has taught him that's wrong. He doesn't know what Jesus taught about how to respect and love others. Instead of rejecting him, you have to be a good example and bring him closer to Jesus."

The professor himself arrived to speak with Audrey.

"Audrey, how are you? Look, if it's difficult for you to have this doctor we can find another one for you."

She said no, that she preferred to continue with the same doctor. And so the doctor came back, a little on the defensive side. Audrey apologized and held out her hand, looking at him with sweetness. The doctor was disconcerted. What had happened to her? From that day on, Audrey was extremely kind to him, intent on recovering lost ground. She prayed for him every day and was docile in his hands. One Sunday, Audrey was watching the Mass on television when the doctor arrived.

"What are you looking at?"

"It's the Mass."

With very simple words, Audrey explained to the doctor that Jesus died for us on the cross and stayed with us in the Eucharist, to give us his body and his blood that he had shed to save us. The doctor looked at her with admiration, although he didn't understand too much of what he was hearing. She continued with this doctor for several months until she had to go into the sterile bubble. When the moment to leave the sterile bubble arrived, she insisted that they send the same doctor to take care of her.

Jerome had noticed that from a very young age Audrey would avert her eyes from indecent advertisements when they were out on the street. Granny remembers an occasion when they were watching television together in the hospital and a yogurt commercial with a scantily dressed girl came on. Audrey said, "Poor girl. Granny, let's pray for her." And they prayed together for the unknown model.

Audrey suffered from something worse than physical pain at night. Stuck in her bed, trapped, she couldn't help hearing, seeing, and feeling the invasion of the "un-elegant." The staff left the door open and kept watch from outside. So much light! Nights are difficult in the hospital, both for the patients and for the staff. Tiredness, sensitivity...one eats, listens to music, gossips, criticizes, jokes, flirts. Those giggles, those jokes, those coarse comments, the loose, frivolous laughter.... Audrey prayed to Jesus on her pillow: "Help them, forgive them, protect me."

uncle Mick

Before entering the hospital, Audrey prayed for her Uncle McLean, her mother's youngest brother, whom the family affectionately nicknamed "Mick." He had spent a month in Cheshire, Connecticut, at the seminary of the Legionaries of Christ to see if he had a priestly vocation. Audrey prayed for him to "find the right path." After Cheshire and after a few months with his brother Alexander in Hollywood, he spent a year with the Oblates of Blessed Virgin Mary in Boston, still searching.

At Maillot, Audrey was given the news. A letter had arrived saying that McLean had left the seminary. She understood that his superiors had told him that he did not have a vocation. Seated on the steps to the house, next to her grandmother, Audrey commented with indignation, "They can't say that."

From then on, the little girl prayed for him more insistently. After a few months, McLean moved back to Chicago to continue his studies. Audrey kept praying. She never doubted his vocation.

Granny had taught her to knit, so in the hospital, she decided to knit him a scarf as a Christmas present. There she was in bed, barefoot and in her pajamas, knitting away at top speed. She was worried about finishing on time. The scarf gradually grew. The scarf was perfectly knitted but, as often happens with beginning knitters, it came out wider on the ends and narrower in the middle. But Audrey finished her work very satisfied, just before

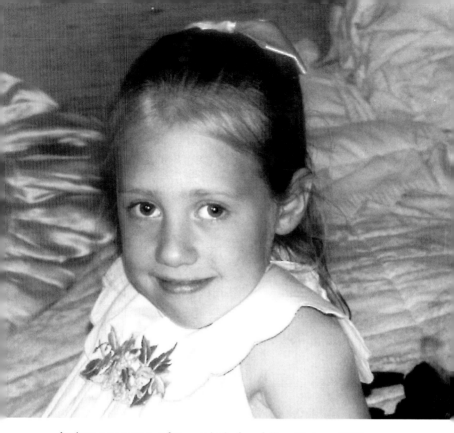

Audrey, age seven, a few weeks before falling ill, June 1990

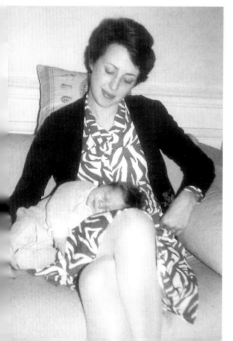

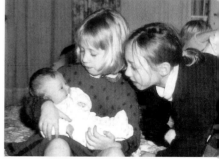

(Left) Audrey, three weeks old, with Mummy

(Above) Aline and Audrey, enjoying Béatrice, the new baby

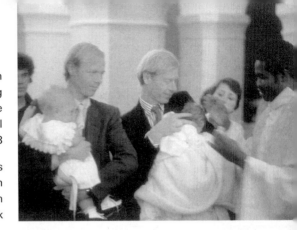

Jerome and his twin brother Marc holding Audrey and Antoine during the baptismal ceremony, April 1993

(Below) Audrey as a toddler sitting on Papa's lap during an outing at the park

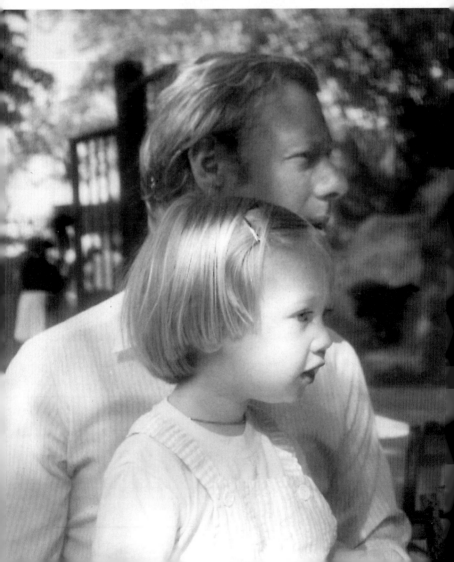

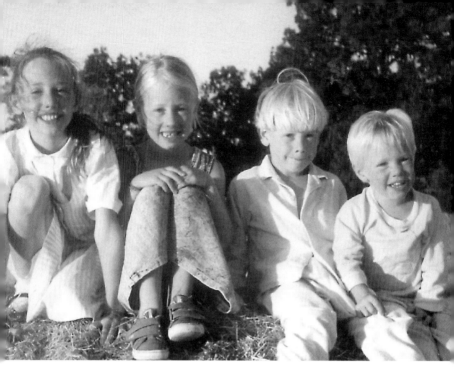

(Above) Aline, Audrey, Henry, and Grégoire, July 1990, playing in their PJs on a haystack in Normandy, a few days before the leukemia is diagnosed

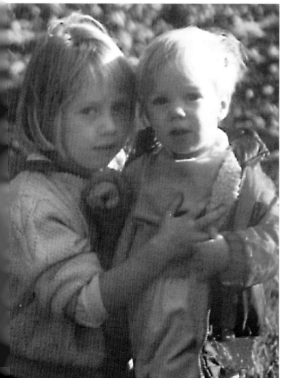

(Left) Audrey with her little protégé Grégoire, October 1988

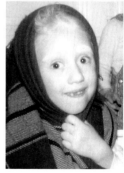

(Above) Audrey loved to scare people with her disguise of an old woman

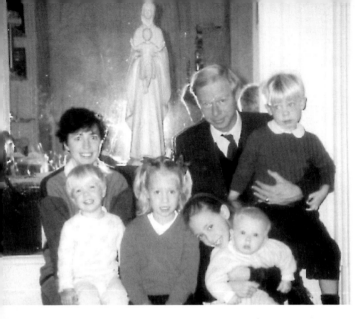

(Left) Audrey gathered the family for night prayers in front of their statue of Mother Mary

(Below) Audrey in the pool, her favorite summer activity, early July 1990

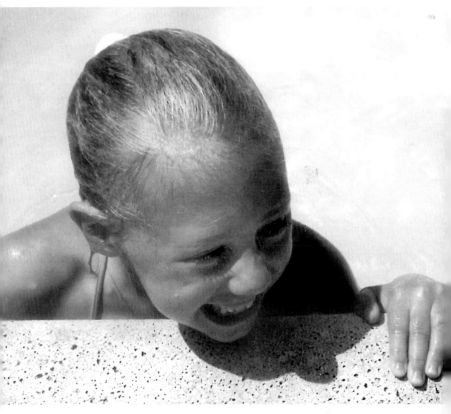

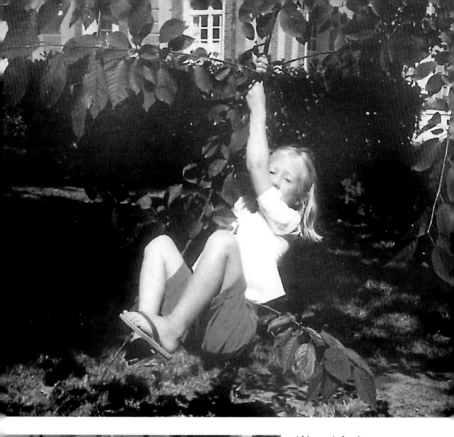

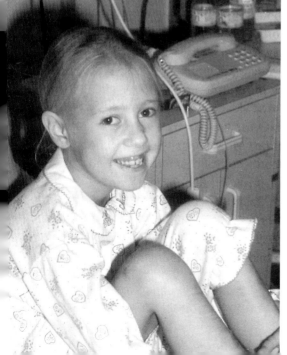

(Above) Audrey enjoyed any physical games, such as swinging and climbing trees in the garden at Maillot

(Left) Audrey posing for her father at the Robert Debré hospital, November 1990

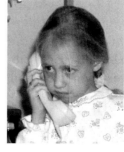

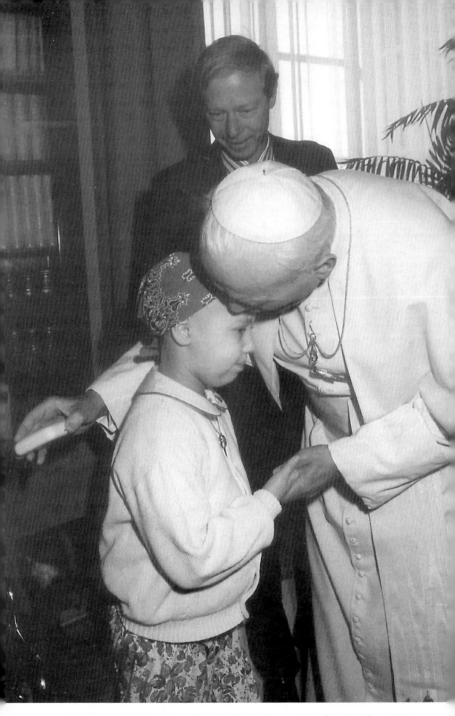

Audrey speaks "in private" with His Holiness John Paul II, May 1991

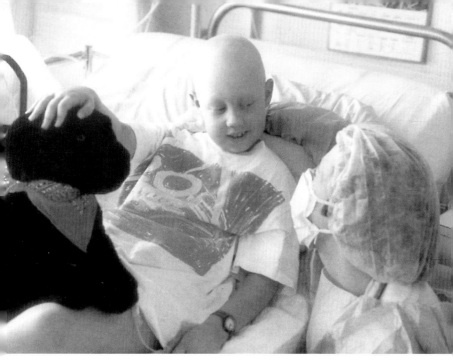

(Above) Audrey and Mummy in the sterile "bubble," reunited for the first time since the transplant, April 1991 (Below) Audrey, in Rome, is blessed by Fr Marcial Maciel, L.C., founder of the congregation of the Legion of Christ, May 1991

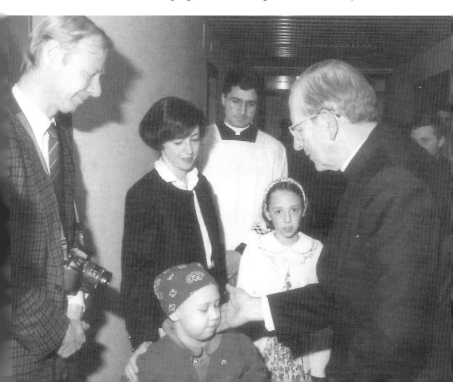

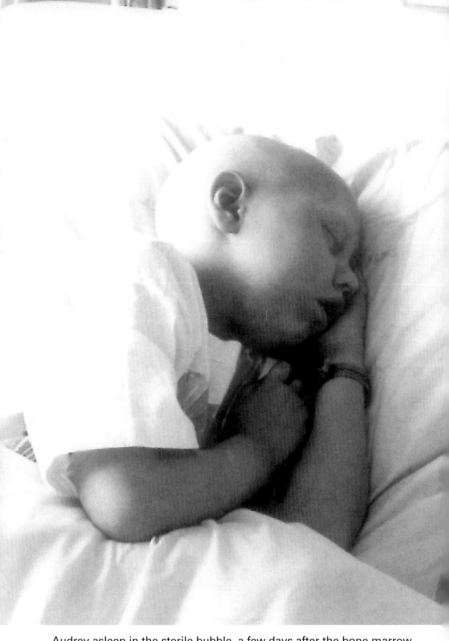

Audrey asleep in the sterile bubble, a few days after the bone marrow transplant, March 1991

Christmas. At the end, she stretched it out to see how it looked. What a surprise! It was bigger than she was. She laughed with pleasure, thinking of the expression on Uncle Mick's face when he would see it. It was a big secret. While she was knitting, she was dreaming of seeing her uncle celebrate Mass, imagining him with the chasuble and praying for him to Jesus and Mary.

christmas

People were hastening to leave the store. It was late.

"Is it this one, Madame? You know we have to close up soon...."

"Yes, I know; please, excuse me. It's the doll they've been advertising on TV so much."

Lillian crossed off another item on her wrinkled bit of paper: it was the list that Audrey had given her. She had to finish her shopping as quickly as possible. The shop clerks had no idea what it meant to prepare for Christmas with a little girl in the hospital. So many presents....

By the shop windows of Printemps, the passers-by were lit up by the street lamps.

At this hour, the dolls in the shop windows no longer moved. Lillian didn't even notice. For her, this Christmas was not like the others. Audrey hadn't said anything, nor had she complained. Yet it was obvious that it was very hard for her not to be at home for Christmas.

The family had prepared a nativity scene, a "crèche," in a little room adjacent to Jerome and Lillian's. The children referred to the room as the chapel: here was the statue of Mother Mary, here they kept their little religious ornaments and books, and here they gathered for the night prayer that had become a tradition—an even more important tradition now that everyone prayed for Audrey. The crèche was made up of little clay figurines and decorated with moss. There was a little bridge and a cave made of wood and straw, and a little lamb for each child. On the first of December, they gave the starting signal. It was a race! On the 24th, before midnight, all of the little lambs had to be in the cave at the feet of the Child Jesus. Your little lamb advanced one step if you did a good deed. Lillian made a little "crèche" for Audrey in her hospital room, and her little lamb was there too.

She and Lillian were watching television together.

"Mummy, look. That's the doll that I thought of for Beatrice— the one that crawls and says, "*Maman*," and turns its head."

The commercials continued and Lillian took note. Audrey knew exactly what each one would like to receive. Between the two of them, they had made a list of one present for each member of the family.

A few days before Christmas, Audrey said, "Mummy, go to my room. Open my drawer and you will see. What you find there is for Christmas."

In the drawer, Lillian found a mountain of well-wrapped presents for the whole family with Audrey's little lettering on each one: "From Audrey for Mami." "From Audrey for Beatrice." In October, when she was home, she had chosen a present for each member of the family from among all her things. For Brigitte, her godmother; for Aline; for Henry. And for Mummy—what a secret! What a delight! Without her mother's knowledge, and with the help of her aunt Beatrice, she had made her a precious necklace. She also prepared some simple gifts, some handmade crafts she had made with the help of the "Pink Ladies." For Grégoire, she made a napkin holder in the shape of Père Noël and a little wooden airplane made out of clothespins.

On Christmas Day, the whole family received a personal gift from Audrey, including the nanny whom Audrey had never even met. Uncle McLean, very intrigued, unwrapped a rather large package and pulled out a piece of red, white, and green wool.

"A scarf!"

Lillian explained that Audrey had made it for him in the hospital. Mick, very moved, noticed the shape. It was wider at the two ends.

"It looks like a stole!"

The scarf stirred up his most intimately held ideals. Months later, McLean was still feeling the arrow of his niece Audrey, the little angel who protected him.

I Am on The Cross

On December 20, there was an unexpected relapse. This time, they thought she would die. To save her, they gave her a dose of chemotherapy that was at the very limits of what she could bear. They feared heart failure, and Lillian didn't want to leave her alone at night. The room had only Audrey's bed, the television, a night table, and an armchair. There was nothing provided for mothers, nothing to be able to sleep on in the same room with the patient. The first night, she tried to get some sleep in the armchair the best she could. Audrey was doing very poorly; she had a high fever and was vomiting frequently. The pain was more intense than ever. It was a night of combat, one of those nights that seems like it will never end. At the end, dawn...sunrise...clarity. Lillian had fallen asleep in the last hours, and now she awakened with a start. Audrey had been awake for hours. Her little voice and her smile:

"How are you, Mummy? Did you sleep well?"

These were the first words of a girl who, badly wounded, had once again recovered from a battle with death.

The next day, Brigitte came to spend the night with her. She suffered seeing Audrey suffer; the chemotherapy was torturing her. She no longer had any saliva, and her eyelids were stuck to her eyes. Her bones hurt her very much, and she no longer had the strength even to cry. The hours of the night went by, and from the armchair Brigitte heard Audrey repeat, slowly, over and over again: "I am on the cross. I am on the cross." The closed eyes, the sweat, the gesture: Gethsemane.

Rome, January 1991

"*Se nota, se siente, el Papa está presente!*" "*Se nota, se siente, los legionarios están presentes.*"

"You can see it, you can feel it: the Pope is here!" "You can see it, you can feel it, the Legionaries are here."

On December 28th, the papal audience. On the 31st, the Angelus. On January 1st, the solemn Mass dedicated to Mary, Mother of God. On the 3rd, in St. Peter's Basilica, a great multitude gathered together. Many families from Mexico, from the United States, and from Spain, Ireland, and Brazil were present. Why so many people? The Pope was going to ordain sixty Legionary priests. The Legion and Regnum Christi were celebrating the 50th anniversary of the foundation of the order.

On January 3, 1941, a young seminarian from Cotija de la Paz, a small Mexican town lost in the beautiful hills of Michoacán, launched himself on a great adventure. Today, he was presenting sixty of his Legionary sons to be ordained priests of Christ. It was an historic day. Among those seated in the basilica, one could see the blond head of Jerome with four of his children at his side, each blonder than the last. *Qu'il y a du monde!* (How many people there are!)

Father Pierre had filled a bus with French people, including Jerome and his children, and had taken them to Rome. They were the first families and members of the Regnum Christi lay movement in France, and they came to participate in the event and go on a pilgrimage. Each one knew Jerome was asking for Audrey's cure, whispering his prayer in those holy places: between the stones, among the ruins, in the tombs of the apostles and martyrs. Without Lillian and Audrey, he had come with three goals: to take care of the children, to help Father Pierre, and to meet the Pope—in order to ask him to pray for Audrey.

Saint Peter's Basilica was packed. The children were gazing at everything. A monsignor in a violet cassock and a surplice walked with elegance, showing the lectors where to seat themselves.

"And these children—so far forward and in the front row? Ah, they are going to bring up the gifts."

"And where are the new priests?" asked Henry.

"They haven't come out yet. They are in silence. They've been in silence a whole week, praying and preparing themselves for their ordination."

Grégoire began to climb down from his seat.

"Papa, pee-pee."

"But, son! Can't you wait?"

Jerome looked around. Swiss guards, monsignors all over the place, people who still didn't have seats. This was going to be difficult. He got up his courage and took Grégoire in his arms, pushing his way through a veritable obstacle course: ladies with long coats, nuns that pushed, children chasing each other in the corridor, a monsignor with a buttoned cassock and a red sash.

"Bonjour, Monseigneur!"

The Legionary choir was practicing the entrance song, "I will give them a sign...." Grégoire's little-boy voice floated out from amidst the barricades and the huge pillars of the basilica:

"Papa, look at the little angel! It's so fat!"

"Yes, Grég."

He looked for the exit and found two guards. A little smile.

"Excuse me, my little boy wants to go to the bathroom."

"Prego, avanti." ("Please, go ahead.")

Further on, another Swiss Guard was very serious.

"Pardon me, we'll make sure to return right away. It's the bathroom—for the little one."

He checked their tickets.

"Va bene, fatte presto." ("Fine, go quickly.")

Finally, the passageway. On their left, they passed in front of the equestrian statue of Constantine.

It was January, four o'clock in the afternoon and bitterly cold. They climbed the stairs to enter into the public restrooms and Jerome took some money out of his wallet. An unsmiling, fat lady, wearing glasses and a bulky overcoat and scarf, was seated at the entrance. Fortunately, the return was faster. Aline's face lit up upon seeing them.

"Here, here!"

Finally, they were seated. The atmosphere began to warm up with vibrant, young voices practicing their songs. More lights began to turn on. The Swiss Guard had closed the passageways up to the altar. Soon, everything would begin.

"Papa, I want to go to the bathroom."

"Ah, no, Grégoire. Not again."

"Papa, yes. Please."

"Grégoire, absolutely not."

"Papa, I *have* to."

Jerome seized Grégoire and marched off with him to the bathroom at a fast pace, furious. They crossed the central nave of the basilica and went towards the exit. Grégoire, bouncing along in his father's arms, didn't make even a peep. He was a little frightened, a little shocked, at his father's reaction. Once again, the alley, the gust of cold air, the little stairway, the fat lady, and the coins. And then they headed back, Grégoire walking and stumbling with his hand in Papa's hand. Jerome became more calm, saying to himself, "Why get angry? He's just a child. We're going to see the Pope."

Just as they turned a corner, they saw a familiar face in the central portico.

"What a surprise!"

"Jerome! My goodness! This little creature is yours?"

"Yes, there are five of them."

It was Colonel Aloïs, an old friend of Jerome's who was in the Swiss Guard. Jerome told him about Audrey.

"Listen, you don't know how much I would like to meet the Pope and ask him to pray for our intentions."

Jerome gave him the photograph of Audrey, smiling in her flowered pajamas, with the prayer on the back.

"In truth, it will be a little difficult. I can't promise you anything. Give me your phone number and I'll call you tomorrow afternoon."

Jerome couldn't believe it. This seemed like a miracle. He walked away in a daze, without noticing anything more than the crowds, the reflections, and the music.

"To be able to go to a private Mass with the Pope, and for it to happen just out of the blue..." He kissed Grégoire. "My son, you're fantastic!" Grégoire was clueless.

The next day, around four in the afternoon, the phone rang.

"Listen, Monsignor Stanislaw said yes, but only three people can come. Be in front of the Portone di Bronzo tomorrow morning at 6:30."

Jerome didn't have time to think. This was truly incredible. He had to prepare himself well; tomorrow he would be speaking to the Pope.

The children ran in zigzags around the blocks of granite. They passed by the Colonnade in front of St. Peter's. Jerome kept a vigilant eye on the children and on their shoelaces; with the other eye, he scanned the horizon for his quarry: red or a biretta.[4] At that moment, the word "clergy" meant "run for him!" and then plead:

"Your Excellency, please, would you be so kind as to give this photo to the Holy Father? It's very important. It's my daughter who is sick with leukemia. Please."

---

4. A "biretta" is the small round skullcap worn by cardinals, monsignors, and bishops.

He had managed to get one of these photos to Monsignor Stanislaw Dziwisz, the Holy Father's personal secretary. The Pope signed it, the Monsignor gave it to a Legionary, and a few days later it arrived back in Jerome's hands.

Brigitte, Aline, and Jerome attended the private Mass. They were seated on the dark purple cushions in the pews of the Holy Father's private chapel, following the Mass with wonder. Jerome stood very attentively, missing none of the Holy Father's movements.

At the end, the Pope greeted each one of the attendees with kindness and interest. When he came over to them, Jerome quickly told him the reason for their visit. The Holy Father inclined his head a little, lifted his eyebrows; listened. His gaze looked far away, turned serious and profound. He took the photograph of Audrey and observed it intently.

"Audrey, Audrey. Yes, we will pray for her."

They returned to Paris. What was going to happen? Their hands were full of graces received, but there was also an emptiness and the most absolute uncertainty. Fear and hope. Faith and love. The children played on the bus while the others slept. Father Pierre thought. Jerome kept to himself in smiles and tears. *Cristus vincit, Cristus regnat, Cristus imperat.*[5]

---

5. Christ conquers, Christ reigns, Christ rules.

☙

victim of love

"Oh, Jesus, it's hardly possible for me to tell all the little souls of the ineffableness of your condescension… I beg you to cast your gaze upon a great number of small souls… I beg you to choose a legion of small victims worthy of your LOVE!"

ST. THÉRÈSE OF LISIEUX

winter

Audrey's soul continued to increase in beauty even as her body was consumed by illness. There are things that one never gets used to, and for Audrey, the hospital was one of those things. Of course, the instruments, the colors, the clothes, the sounds, and the rolling of the beds down the corridors all became familiar to her. But she continued to feel like a little girl hidden away in a forest of adults. A little girl in that huge building with its seemingly infinite number of floors, units, areas, rooms, patients, and shift numbers. A little girl moved from place to place by unknown hands to unfamiliar places, and hooked up to machines that were enormous, noisy, full of wires and cables, with needles and bright lights. The world of a hospital is very impressive, even more so for a child.

Some days were good days; others were very bad. She wasn't able to take the quantity of pills she needed to take every day. The irritation of the chemotherapy made the pills difficult to swallow, and their content made her throw up. But she wanted to keep on participating in life. Mummy had given her a guitar for Christmas—to make up for the lack of a piano! And so, helpless, weak, she enthusiastically undertook the task of learning a new instrument. From time to time, she saw a teacher who came to give lessons to the children. She wanted to do her schoolwork more often, but it was not always possible. Audrey made an heroic effort every time she tried to get up out of her bed to go to the little table in her room to do some work. She felt powerless. She spent a few moments in a room prepared with toys to share with the other sick children, but it was not always possible to go. She continued going over her verbs with Mami on some Wednesdays.

In the moments of greater calm and in those of greater pain, day by day she was uniting within herself, in an embrace of oblation, the most human with the most divine. Audrey offered... and offered herself. This became clear, and eloquently so, when they gave her spinal taps and myelograms.[1] Whether they were extracting spinal fluid with a syringe in order to study it or introducing substances into her spinal fluid, it required injections into the spinal column. To remove a sample of bone marrow also required an extremely painful injection. Her bones ached all the time now. It is not difficult to imagine the fear that these injections would create in a child; they were real moments of torture. In a children's hospital, the doctors must know how to act on these occasions. They have to take the patient by surprise and not give him too much time to react and defend himself. It's better if he doesn't recognize the instruments (if it's not the first time), and it's better if his family members are not around. It was a vividly painful experience, and for a child, those were minutes of terror. For the doctors, it was a disagreeable, but necessary procedure. Regardless, Audrey flatly refused to be treated in this way. No. She wanted them to warn her before giving her those injections. One day they had trapped her by surprise, alone and without Mummy. What a humiliation! What a feeling of despair! You overcome the fear later, if you can. No! She told her grandmother and mentioned it to Lillian.

"Mummy, when they are going to do that to me, I want them to tell me first. I want to prepare myself, and I also want you to be with me."

They fought for this permission.

"You see, she's a girl who is a little special. I would like to be there to support her. Please, everything will go well."

The nurses didn't understand and were bothered by the request. The doctors doubted; they didn't believe that Lillian

---

1. A spinal tap is a puncture into the lower region of the spinal cord. It may involve the withdrawal of spinal fluid for analysis, the injection of dye for X-ray imaging, or the administration of anesthesia or medication. A myelogram is the withdrawal of some bone marrow for analysis. It usually is taken from the sternum or the lower back bones.

would be able to go through with it calmly. But in the end, they agreed. Lillian would have special permission to be at her daughter's side for each injection. Face mask, sterilized bonnet, sterilized overshoes—she was dressed like a surgeon.

An injection like that was something to live freely; it was something to suffer freely. From December until the moment she entered the sterilized bubble, they gave her the injection every week, always in the morning. And they warned her: one hour of warning.... Audrey would then recollect herself; she would go into the desert, seek Jesus, and pray. They would come into her room, and lay her facedown.

"Father, save me from this hour. But not as I will, but as you will."

Lillian was at her side. She put her face next to Audrey's.

"Mummy, let's offer it for Uncle Mick, for Papa so that he'll stop smoking, and for the nuns in Bordeaux who have no vocations."

Audrey took a breath, and a tear rolled down her cheek. Her body contracted. She breathed in short gasps, with effort. She had to control the pressure. Had to control her heart. Here there were no painkillers or tranquilizers. Audrey and Lillian repeated the prayer. Slowly.

"For Uncle...Mick. For Papa...for the nuns and the vocations...."

She repeated it more hurriedly, doing whatever she could to endure the pain. The fifteen minutes lasted an eternity. It was finished. Her muscles relaxed. She lay there, her body drained and exhausted. She couldn't move. And if it was a spinal tap, an intense headache followed. She would spend the rest of the day prostrate, crushed, worn down, like someone who survived a beating. Lillian left the room. She was bent down under the pressure; her knees were weak. It was too tense, too hard. It had been a moment of prayer.

At the end of January, Audrey received a surprise visit. It was her friend Hector, the consecrated man! She blushed a little to be seen like that, in bed, in her pajamas. Hector was struck upon seeing her. She was just as sweet, just as joyful, but more calm. And her gaze…if before it had said much, now it held who knows how many divine secrets. Hector told her what he had been doing lately. He had been in Poland. How many young people there were to invite to work for Christ! Soon he would be going to England. Audrey listened very attentively. The day after his visit, Lillian telephoned Hector. He was surprised; Lillian had never called him before. That morning, as it happened, she had arrived at the hospital and had accompanied Audrey to her injection. Audrey had wanted to offer it for him. At the end, she said, "Mummy, I offered it for Hector, and it hurt me much less."

From that day on, Hector felt especially protected by Audrey in his vocation. He kept her photograph in his agenda in order to keep it near him and carry it with him always.

Later that week, a nurse asked, "What's all that noise?" It was Audrey, entertaining herself with the song *La Bamba* turned up at full volume. Hector had left her the tape of the Legionaries of Christ's orchestra as a gift, and it brought back very good memories.

The month of February arrived, a very hard month for Audrey. The doctors had to prepare her for the bone marrow transplant. It was the only solution that medicine could offer in order to help her body produce healthy white blood cells. They would have to destroy Audrey's own marrow almost totally, leaving only enough so that she could survive. The doses of chemotherapy were going to push her body's resistance to the limit.

With all of that, Audrey found out that they were organizing a little costume party for the sick children, and she wouldn't miss out. She asked them to disguise her as a clown. There she appeared in her wheelchair, more disguised than ever, covered from head to toe, wearing a hat and a smock, with a red nose and painted eyes.

Before the transplant, they would have to subject her to three days of radiation therapy, and following that, she would have to enter a sterile bubble. There were only two hospitals in Paris equipped for radiation therapy, and they would have to transport her with the greatest care, since she was now practically without immune defenses, to a different hospital. Radiation therapy.... In the midst of her pain they stretched her out and smeared her with a strong-smelling product, as if she were a chicken ready to roast. Then they fastened suction cups and some rubber bands with sticky plaster to her and drew marks on her with indelible ink. If only it were possible, just for a minute, to feel Mummy's arms! Even so, Audrey always remained calm, always serene. She didn't show fear, worry, or discouragement. Sometimes she would have to keep absolutely still for long periods of time, up to forty-five minutes. It frightened Lillian to see how quiet and still she was. It also struck the doctors and solved quite a few problems for them.

They put her in position.

"Don't move at all."

They went behind the window. From inside the cabin, they pushed buttons, pulled levers, activated switches. The noise was long and heavy. The nurse was prepared: if a child moved, he would have to be held firmly, strapped into position, and fastened to the table. The session began. By means of the open audio communication system used with the patient, they could hear a keen little voice. There were a few ironic faces among the specialists.

"She's singing to the Virgin Mary."

Yes, Audrey kept herself entertained by singing. *"Tu es là, au cœur de ma vie.... Si le Père vous appelle.... Le Seigneur fait pour moi des merveilles...."*[2] They were the songs she sang in the car with

---

2. "You are there, in the heart of my life.... If the Father calls you.... The Lord has done great things for me...."

Aline, on the way to Maillot; they were the songs they sang in bed to get to sleep. She paused a moment to remember the words and began the verse again. Then she would recite Hail Marys and all the vocal prayers that she knew. In this way, time went by a little more quickly. The doctor interrupted her through the microphone:

"Very good, Audrey. Your song is very pretty, but now we are going to turn you over, facedown."

Lillian accompanied her to this new hospital, and they installed Audrey in a sterile room that even Mummy could not enter. Then Lillian and Audrey would return to Robert Debré hospital in a special ambulance that was completely protected. Two motorcycle police would go in front in order to clear the way through the traffic.

Before the radiotherapy, Jerome and Lillian asked for very special permission for Audrey's brothers and sisters to come see her, just for a moment, just for five minutes. They were allowed to come. Audrey prepared herself; she was thrilled. She hadn't seen them for four months. An eternity! She had hidden caramel candies for Grégoire and Beatrice in the drawer of her night table.

"Beatrice, look in the drawer, look in the drawer!"

Audrey watched her baby sister with intense pleasure while she stretched out her little arm to open it and then ran back to Mummy with her hands full of candies.

Transplant

An icy wind blew. With her overcoat and scarf wrapped around her, Aline talked with her friends about the trip to Rome.

"We showed him the photograph of Audrey, and he said he would pray for her."

Audrey: her great hero, her invincible sister. There was an

uncertainty in her voice when she said her name. The future appeared so far away; so distant from her reality. The here and now was all she had.

"Now they are going to take blood samples and do tests on me and my brother Henry. It's for a bone marrow transplant for Audrey. One of us is going to give her our bone marrow."

On March 1st, Audrey was put into the sterile bubble. It consisted of a bed surrounded by a wall of clear plastic curtains. It was completely sterilized and isolated from the exterior. No one could enter or touch Audrey. The only way to touch her was by putting one's hands in special gloves that Audrey could touch from inside. The bed was placed in a small glass room. Only the doctors and nurses could enter this glass room. Even to be on this other side of the bubble, special permission was needed.

And so Lillian got permission. She was covered from head to toe in sterile garments, as required. Through some microphones, the patient could speak to the person on the other side of the glass, and from that other side, one could see and accompany the person inside. Audrey would hold up the objects that she wanted to show. She would be there for six weeks...without touching Mummy.

The date for the transplant was set for Friday, the 8th of March. Audrey had been left almost totally without defenses. A catheter continuously administered what medicine she needed. Besides that, she was connected to tubes for medicine, for intravenous feeding, and for the blood and bone marrow transfusions.

What was left of her? Suspended between heaven and earth, she lived as a beggar. Her blood was not her blood. She had been abandoned into the hands of men. With her child's soul and her child's heart, Audrey was pouring herself out for sinners and for the sanctification of souls.

At the Robert Debré Hospital, there was a closed-circuit television that made the children participants in the life of the hospital, which put on special programs for and about them. Audrey wanted to go on television, too. She wanted to explain to all the children about the two types of catheters that exist. She had had both of them, and wanted to explain how they were attached and how they felt, so that once they saw that she had used them and that "nothing had happened to her," the children who needed them would no longer be afraid to have them implanted. There was also a hospital newspaper. Basing her work on a well-known tune, Audrey wrote a song about her illness for publication. Nobody could deny that his little girl could laugh at anything, even her own shadow.

One day, Audrey couldn't see anything. All around her was black. She didn't scream. She didn't cry. She didn't say anything. Just like every day, Lillian came to visit her, and they spent the day together, talking. Audrey continued on without being able to see anything at all, but still she said nothing. The television was on. Afterwards, they prayed together. Audrey even dialed the telephone to call home. She said nothing about her eyes. The next day came. Audrey was in the midst of reading a series of adventure stories, but today she asked Mummy to read the book out loud to her. Afterwards, Lillian proposed that they play a game, but Audrey asked her to keep on reading. Lillian read to her almost the whole day.

Before leaving, Lillian asked her, "Would you like me to turn on *Little House on the Prairie?*"

"Better not. My eyes hurt a little when I watch TV."

Lillian had noticed nothing. She could only see Audrey through the plastic curtains that surrounded Audrey's bed. She observed her intently. Now she suddenly realized that Audrey couldn't see. Deep down she felt a mixture of tears and indignation, with a stab of pain. The doctors told Lillian that the loss of sight was probably temporary, although they weren't sure. It was a consequence of the new chemotherapy treatment they had administered. Audrey spent days without even mentioning the pain in her eyes or her blindness. She behaved so simply and naturally that Lillian almost forgot that her daughter couldn't see. She continued to receive her daily phone call from Audrey in the hospital, and it didn't occur to her to wonder how Audrey had managed to dial the number, which was quite long: four numbers to get the outside line, other numbers for the area code, and then the eight numbers to reach home. Thanks be to God, after ten days she regained her sight. Lillian wondered, though, if her eyes were exactly the same beautiful blue that they had been....

With all that, Audrey remained the same: only God and her guardian angel know how she managed, as a new arrival to the sterile bubble, to fill a surgical glove with water and hang it on top of the door. A nurse, upon entering, received an unexpected shower...and a rather cold one at that!

Henry

The 8th of March drew near. It was the chosen date for the bone marrow transplant. The donor was her brother Henry.

It was Lent. In the chapel of the house, on Jules Verne Street, they had put a crown of thorns, a little basket full of pretty paper flowers, and another empty basket. The children would write an effort they intended to make on a little piece of paper and put it in the empty basket. If they fulfilled it, they could take a flower and put it on the crown. By Easter Sunday, the crown of thorns would be transformed into a real crown of flowers, and they would put it on the head of the Baby Jesus that they had in the hallway. All of this was Audrey's idea. She was extremely conscious of the need to prepare her crown for eternal life.

Aline was conscious as well. She had left her little paper in the sacrifice basket. "I am going to offer my hair for Audrey." Lillian had been rather surprised at the explanation Aline had given when she asked her to cut her hair. It was long, and Aline loved it.

"Mummy, I want you to cut my hair very short. Then, when Audrey's hair starts to grow back, I will trim mine little by little so that we can have it the same length."

Now Henry had to save his sister. When the doctors spoke with Jerome and Lillian about the possibility of a transplant, Jerome commented to Lillian that it would be marvelous if they could choose Henry. It would be the most eloquent sign of reconciliation between him and Audrey. The doctors did the tests to see which sibling's marrow was most compatible with Audrey's, and the parents had no say in the decision. The doctors finally proposed the male as the donor because they thought it might help if the donor and Audrey were not of the same sex.

It was very beautiful. Henry was already five, and after the illness had struck, he had done everything he could for his sister. Now he had his great opportunity: he would suffer for her to save her.

Audrey was profoundly touched by the news that her brother was going to be operated on to give her his marrow, and once again, she felt sorry for having been exasperated with him so many times. They brought Henry to the operating room. In the bed, he looked everywhere, observing, waving at people. He was very serene; it was all for his sister. In that moment, he felt that his salvific love could have conquered all the dragons on earth.

It was a very important day both for Audrey and for the staff at the hospital. The operation would be a matter of one or two hours. They would extract the marrow from the boy, analyze it quickly in the laboratory, and bring it up to the fifth floor. Those who were present were paying close attention to every move. Audrey still couldn't see.

"Now we are putting in your brother's marrow."

Before the boy woke up, Audrey was already receiving his marrow through the catheter. Some floors below, Henry was rapidly recuperating from his heroic exploit. There was such satisfaction in his gaze…he felt strong, like a conqueror. Mami accompanied Audrey, while Lillian was with Henry.

Audrey kept asking: "Mami, has Henry woken up yet? Mami, is it hurting Henry? Mami, why don't you go keep Henry company for a while? He must be alone and frightened. He doesn't know much about hospitals…."

"Happy Birthday to you, Happy Birthday to you!" It was March 18th, and Audrey was now eight. She was recuperating from the bone marrow transplant. It had been a while since they had last given her chemotherapy, and she seemed happy; she felt less uneasy. It would be a very unusual birthday. Few could come to visit her, and if they did, they had to greet her from behind the glass. Her bubble was filled with presents—all sterilized! Papa arrived with a radiant face. He would have liked to present her with a black Labrador, but it was impossible because of the circumstances. Now he saw her in her bed, laughing and hugging an enormous black stuffed dog, a gift from her cousins.

"It's Drum!"

And that was not all. She also received a very important visit. The cameramen from Channel Plus came to film her. Yes, she was going to be on television as part of a documentary program entitled *Twenty-Four Hours in the Hospital*. The Robert Debré Children's Hospital was brand-new, and people wanted to know about it. They interviewed Audrey in her bubble, and she was delighted to take advantage of the opportunity to encourage other children with her example and show her joy in the midst of suffering. The cameraman really did spend twenty-four hours in the hospital. He came and went, filming Audrey at long intervals so that he could choose the best shots afterwards. Curiously enough, a close-up of a picture of St. Thérèse of the Child Jesus appeared twice, even in the final edited version. The cameraman thought that it was the Virgin Mary, but Audrey immediately cleared up that confusion, telling him the whole story of the saint.

Suffering had not changed her personality in the least. Even in the bubble, she had not lost her inclination to the life of the circus. She continued putting on plays with her sterilized dolls, and colored with her sterilized crayons. It was here that she made the drawings of her future career: the circus, Drum, and Carmel.

Her parents gave her a present—a little electronic keyboard. On the day of her birthday, the professor came to visit her in her bubble.

"Audrey, play something for me on your little piano."

There, with her dressing gown, her swollen face, and without hair, she immediately turned on the keyboard, chose a sound, and played "ding-dong, ding-dong." She had chosen an ambulance siren! The professor was a little taken aback by her promptness to tease him and didn't know what to say.

She followed the movements of the nurses with her eyes and was part of everything that happened with the staff. Not one of them escaped her. And she prayed for them. She continued praying for the other sick children. She enjoyed making them laugh with that red clown's nose and by balancing Drum on her head. Of course, those too were sterilized.

Just down the hall, there was a little black boy who was four years old. Audrey was worried because she knew that they were waiting for a donor for the little boy, and it was difficult to find a compatible one. In a kind, but businesslike way, she called for the professor's assistant. He was a very important doctor, and he was black, like her little companion.

"Sir, this boy across the hall doesn't have a bone marrow donor. Couldn't you give him yours?"

The kind doctor smiled and explained that it wasn't that simple....

Lillian shared with Audrey a case that Uncle Marc, Jerome's twin, had told her about. It was the case of a little boy from Bordeaux named Pierre. He had a very serious illness, and the doctors needed to operate on him. His parents were good Christians and were in the Emmanuel Movement. Nevertheless, it was a sad case, because he had rebelled strongly against Jesus. Pierre was angry with Jesus and didn't love him anymore. Audrey felt great sorrow at this news and began to pray with all her strength. She would offer many things for him. After a while, they told her, "Look what happened to this boy. It turned out that on the day of his operation, just before he entered the operating room, he called his mother and asked her to put his gold chain with his baptismal medal around his neck." Audrey said nothing, but her face lit up completely. Her joy was beyond words.

Her next action was to seize a piece of paper and write this little boy a real "Philippian" epistle: "I am very happy with what has happened…but you have to promise me right now that you will never lose your faith again."

Holy Thursday

Lillian walked down the corridor with rapid steps. Her face was tense, and she was intently focused on the anxious question, *Will it work?* She forced herself to respond with friendliness, in the midst of her exhaustion, to the people who asked her about the results of the transplant: "How is your daughter doing?" There were certain times when it is very bothersome to be asked kind questions. Of course, they didn't mean to be bothersome. But that woman, so dressed up and with such long nails…if she only knew how painful her well-meaning comments were! Nurses that she hadn't seen for weeks were following Audrey's story from a distance, even after having taken care of her for only one or two days. They drew closer, wanting to know. A tall, handsome doctor walked by, his smock unfastened. He strode by with a sporty gait, without stopping, and made a cheerful gesture with his hand as if to say, "Don't worry, lady. Everything will come out fine, just fine."

Lillian thought, *And you? What do you know? God knows. Only God knows.*

The whole staff broke with their monotonous routines to investigate the results of the transplant. The entire ward was awaiting the results. If the transplant succeeded, it would be a success, a real "score" for science—a real feather in the medical team's cap.

And then there were the Tuesday Rosaries. The children didn't know what a transplant was. Jerome kept the families updated as usual. They listened and commented. They didn't understand the procedure very well, but it was obvious to them that this required many prayers. So they began to pray, some standing, leaning against the wall; others seated on the arm of a sofa or on the floor. There were the fathers of families, with their ties and their smart suits, keeping count on their rosaries. There were the mothers with their children half-asleep in their arms.

The children intensified every Hail Mary. They were sure that Audrey would get better. Audrey was a friend of Jesus, a friend of the Virgin Mary; they would cure her. The war broke out in Yugoslavia, and a little boy arrived at the Rosary very determined, saying that he had been told that with the Rosary they were going to be able to stop the bombs. The intention was immediately adopted. That evening, the prayer was particularly fervent. At the end of the Rosary, Jerome, very moved, said warmly to the children:

"Look, children, it's true! Today there is a bomb that didn't fall in Yugoslavia, thanks to your prayers."

There was a stunned silence, and tears shone in the eyes of many of those present.

In the hospital laboratory, the calls came in one after another:

"Any news?"

"Nothing yet."

Lillian parked the car. The churches in Paris were preparing for Holy Week. In the Madeleine, they were putting up an altar of repose for the Blessed Sacrament. A purple cloth next to the altar in Saint Germain des Près said "Convertissez-vous."[3] The organ of Saint Sulpice was practicing Bach's *St. Matthew's Passion*. They were also preparing the procession of the Blessed Sacrament for Holy Thursday; it would go from the banks of the Seine to Notre Dame Cathedral. Paris was full of solemnity. The splendid bells would remain silent until the morning of the Resurrection. Then, Spring would burst into the park of Les Tuileries, in the Park Monceau, in the Boulevard de Malesherbes.

Good Friday.... A whirl of white doctors' coats.... A piece of great news: "She's producing white blood cells, and they're healthy!"

The hospital was filled with euphoria, and there was an atmosphere of resurrection. The nurses congratulated each other. The doctors congratulated each other. The nurses congratulated the doctors. It made everyone so happy! Imprudently happy—science had conquered! The staff had conquered. Audrey had conquered. Her mother, her father, and her family, who had kept her going with so much patience—they had all conquered! Good Friday was also the day on which Jesus conquered sin and death.

Audrey's immune system was becoming stronger, so they allowed Lillian to enter the sterile bubble to spend some time with her. It was a long-awaited moment. After so many long weeks, she could see her a little bit closer. She could not touch her, as she still had to wear her latex gloves and her face mask. But they were together at last, on the same side of the plastic curtain. Lillian wished that time could stop, but it was impossible; besides,

---

3 "...unto dust you will return."

she had to prepare for Easter. On Sunday, there would be a big meal with the whole family. She had to buy chocolate eggs to hide in the garden for the little ones, put special flowers in front of the Virgin, and prepare Beatrice's smocked party dress.

Suddenly, Audrey suffered a stab of great pain. Her face contracted. Her gaze clouded over and her eyes closed. Seated, she put her two hands on her chest and leaned over repeatedly.

"It's my heart, it's my heart!"

With her right thumb, she made the sign of the cross over and over again on the place where it hurt. Then she sank back on her pillows, perfectly still. It had only lasted a few seconds. Lillian was very frightened. She immediately called the nurse, thinking that Audrey was having a heart attack. On the cardiogram, Audrey's heartbeat plunged down, as if she were dead. Lillian looked at her watch: it was exactly 3:00 in the afternoon. Good Friday.

Lillian thought Audrey was dead, but the electrocardiogram kept working. The rhythm was regular again. A nurse came in briskly, interrupting the shock of the mother, who was watching her daughter without daring to touch her. She looked at the cardiogram and then at Lillian's terrified face. "Ma'am, she's sleeping. Why did you call me?"

Lillian looked at her without seeing her. She didn't know what to say. She was confused and very frightened. How to explain it to her? Lillian didn't want to think, but she thought of the passion of Christ. Beyond the success of the transplant, beyond science, beyond the lit up faces of the doctors and nurses, God was asking Audrey for a total union. It was like a warning: "Don't think it has gone your way. She is still mine." Lillian pondered these things in her heart. There was still a long way to go. Audrey was in the hands of God, and she didn't belong to them. He would continue leading Audrey by the way of the cross until the day when she, together with Jesus, would ring the bells of Eternal Joy.

At Home

On April 15, Audrey came out of the sterile bubble to go into a normal room, crossing the hospital corridors in her wheelchair. How long those weeks had been! She smiled and greeted the people she met on the way. It was wonderful to see more people, even though they were only nurses with their little carts in the corridors and elevators. Her eyes looked around at everything with enthusiasm. In her room once more, everything was a big celebration. She had such a desire to play, to laugh, to joke, and she lifted the spirits of everyone who came to visit her. Her hair was starting to grow back, and the hint of an eyebrow could be seen. When her grandmother saw her, tears sprang into her eyes.

Audrey walked around her room with great satisfaction, pleased that Mami could see her walking. Of course, she wanted to study verbs again, and she asked Mami to bring her notebooks for the next visit. She showed up in the little playroom off to the side to play with the other children, and she took up guitar lessons again. One afternoon, Lillian opened the door to find Audrey out of bed, bouncing a ball. "The most beautiful day of my life!" she thought.

Nathalie came to her room every day. She was the physiotherapist, a fun-loving, kind girl whose job was to make Audrey exercise and move her muscles so that they wouldn't atrophy and so she would regain some muscle tone after the long weeks in bed. They did exercises together, playing with the ball.

"Listen, if I hit it ten times in a row, you have to pay me five francs."

"Audrey!" Lillian intervened.

She knew that her daughter wanted to save up in order to buy a real dog, but still, she didn't approve of this "system." Yes, she remembered her daughter at Maillot. Lillian had thought that Audrey was collecting shells in order to paint and decorate them. But it wasn't really for that; what she really wanted was to sell them to her uncles and grandparents to earn money. Lillian gave her permission on the condition that she would not fix the prices. With just one price fix, she could easily leave them all bankrupt. Nathalie laughed. She wasn't much of a believer, but she had to marvel at Audrey.

Jerome and Lillian were starting to see the light at the end of the tunnel. They started to talk about her release from the hospital and make plans. "Let's all go to Lourdes. Yes, we'll all go to Lourdes together as a family, and all our friends can come too. We'll make a pilgrimage of thanksgiving to Our Lady."

In a little house in Versailles, people gathered to pray the Rosary. It was Tuesday. An Easter melody danced on the children's lips, and their hearts were full of hope. They had prayed so much....

"Hail Mary, full of grace."

Audrey came home for a day. The doctors had authorized it before her transfer to a special rehabilitation center where she would spend a few months in a sterile and protected environment until her immune system had totally recovered. The month of May had just begun. When she had left home last fall, the cherry tree in front of the house had let its pink petals fall. Now, the branches shook in a gentle welcome, with the tender green of the tree's miniature leaves.

"Look, Audrey, look!"

A sparrow had just landed on a branch. He had a beak full of little twigs, and he was making his nest. Her room was warm and luminous, and it had the same fragrance as always. A splash of spring sunshine caressed her when she sat on the bed, and the birds were tweeting peacefully. Audrey opened all the drawers and, to her joy, found her clothes. It had been so long since she had worn this outfit, her bathing suit, the flip-flops. She was quite happy, the mistress and lady of her own dwelling. How pleasant it was to be home! The chapel was bursting with flowers for Our Lady.

They returned to the hospital once more. Audrey continued with her exercises, but it seemed that she was not regaining her strength at the expected rate. Lillian found it strange that she would get so tired, but the doctors reassured her:

"Don't worry, it's normal. Remember that she's been in bed for months without moving. She has to go little by little."

But Lillian saw that she was becoming weaker, and the doctors didn't seem to understand what was happening. They insisted to Audrey:

"You have to walk. You have to try."

Lillian obeyed the doctors and forced Audrey to walk up and down the corridors. She didn't know how exhausted her daughter really was. With great difficulty and heroic effort, Audrey told her, "Okay, Mummy, I'll walk. But I'll walk for a seminarian."

She kept St. Thérèse of Lisieux in mind. Sick with tuberculosis and exhausted like her, she had forced herself to walk, and each step had been for a missionary. Audrey walked for a little bit and then said, "Mummy, I'd like to go lie down." It hurt her to be so weak, but she was serene. There were no tears. No protests. No fear.

Relapse

They had planned to discharge her from the hospital on the 12th of May.

"Audrey, before you go, we're going to do a little test just to make sure that you're all well."

Audrey became sad. Once again, that injection…how much it hurt! There was fear in Lillian's soul as well. For some days now, she had felt a deep doubt. She braced herself, praying to God and to Mary. She had to be prepared for whatever the Lord wanted. This time, the injection was especially painful. Would she be able to stand it? Lillian could almost touch her daughter's suffering. Together they had decided to offer it for Papa, for a divorced relative, and for the Poor Clares in Bordeaux. She kept repeating the intentions; her voice was very weak, but she drew strength from deep inside. It was Monday, May 13th, the day of the Virgin of Fatima. Ten years ago on this day, an assassin had attempted to take the life of the Pope.

Lillian arrived home without the strength to think, to suspect—without even a sense of time. In the evening, the professor called. He wanted to see her and her husband the next day, early. Jerome and Lillian understood: it wasn't good news. Lillian's first reaction was to feel a sense of helplessness. It wasn't just that she didn't want to lose her daughter. It was also that she asked herself how she could live without her. She made God so present to the family. It was that spirit, that atmosphere, her interior joy, that special strength she radiated that kept everyone going in the faith.

On the next day, Tuesday, the professor received them. One look said it all: the mystery of human failure. The eminent professor was very put out; he couldn't explain why the transplant hadn't worked. Everything was going fine, and then suddenly, Audrey was in serious condition. The index of malignant cells had grown at a galloping pace. It was recommended to keep Audrey in the hospital. There was nothing that could be done, but she would be taken care of. They would give her transfusions and morphine to lessen the pain during her last…three weeks? There was horror in the eyes of her parents. And right away, faith and abandonment to God. They were offered a small hope: an experimental treatment…. Jerome and Lillian barely had to discuss it before it was decided. They would take Audrey out of the hospital now, take her to Lourdes, and then they would see.

Audrey could only go for three days without a transfusion, so they had to act quickly. It was madness to bring a little girl like that, with no strength, no immunity. The car, the plane, the humidity, the fatigue...but they launched themselves forth. Lillian got instructions from the hospital and filled a duffel bag with sterilized food and medicines. How to administer the morphine when the bone pain became unbearable, how to apply the serum, what to do if she fell into a coma.... Doctors and nurses surrounded her, perplexed. To Lourdes?

Now the girl was in the hands of her parents and the Lord. Jerome got the plane tickets, and Lillian telephoned the whole family.

"The doctors have no more hope. Please pray. Tomorrow, we're going to Lourdes. Come with us, as many as you can."

On Wednesday morning, Lillian came into Audrey's room.

"Audrey, I'm going to take you home."

"But aren't they going to put me in a recovery house?"

Lillian collected her daughter's few belongings and the many medicines.

"No, Audrey. The transplant didn't work. We're going home."

"Are they going to do a second transplant?"

Lillian drew near and gently told her, "We are going to do just what we did in the beginning when you first got sick. Do you remember?"

Audrey understood. "Yes. We are going to live like the birds of the sky. One day at a time."

In her eyes, there was a silent listening, an acceptance. Lillian then told her that they would be going to Lourdes, and her expression changed right away. She became very happy at the prospect of the trip. She would once again be in the beloved place of her first holy Communion! And even better—she would be accompanied by Brigitte, Uncle Marc, Aline, Papa...and the greatest thing of all: Uncle Mick was to fly over from the United States and meet them the next day at the airport.

we're going to Lourdes

"Passengers on Flight #402 to the destination of Tarbes may now begin boarding at Gate Four."

"Look, haven't you seen that girl before?"

"Yes, but where?"

"She was on TV last week. She was in a bubble."

"Ah, yes. The documentary on the children's hospital."

In the airport, word got around. Ladies and some children examined her with curiosity from afar. A pair of young boys came closer to her. With their gaze, they asked permission to draw even closer to Audrey. Jerome smiled. One of the two crouched down. Audrey was sitting in her wheelchair.

"Are you the one who was on TV from the hospital?"

Audrey smiled and looked at the others, enjoying the scene. "Yes."

"Ah, good luck. Hope all goes well."

The boys went away very impressed. Brigitte had come with Johan, her husband. And look who was coming now—Father Pierre! Audrey's face lit up. Her face was tired, but radiant with joy. The little group gathered, and Jerome pushed Audrey's wheelchair; father and daughter were laughing together. Papa was joking, "Yes, ladies and gentlemen! Here comes Audrey, the great television star, accompanied by her inseparable chauffeur."

Audrey burst into laughter. Nobody would have guessed that this girl ran the risk of septicemia. The doctors had given her less than three weeks to live.

The plane lifted off. Below them, Orly became tiny and eventually disappeared under a vast white cloud as big as the horizon. A very nice friend of Father Pierre's would be waiting for them at the Tarbes airport. Then it would be only a half-hour trip to Lourdes, and they would arrive at the hotel.

"Have you had this bad weather for many days?"

"Oh yes, it's always like this in May."

Damp and cold. Very little of the countryside could be seen. The fields were so green. Fog and low clouds lay across the woods, and the trees seemed blanketed in white mist. The children wanted to see the mountains, which are the Lower Pyrenees. Where were they? Already, they could see the Castle of Lourdes, a medieval fortress affixed to the top of a small peak that overlooked the Gave Valley. The narrow streets of the little city were almost empty. Most of the stores and souvenir shops were closed: the Rosary Palace, the House of Bernadette.... The season had not yet begun; in fact, the Virgin stands alone in the grotto for half of the year. Under the porticos, at the entrances to the hospitals, the little blue carts for the invalids were backed up one behind the other. Father Pierre's friend had opened his hotel exclusively for Audrey and her family. It was a very special visit. They got settled. Lillian lay down on the bed and immediately dozed off.

At her side, Audrey, her cousin Antoine, and Aline played a game of cards. Audrey commented in a low voice, thinking that Mummy didn't hear:

"That's funny—I'm the sick one, and Mummy is the one who is sleeping."

The smell of dinner wafted up the stairs. French fries. Audrey was a little disappointed; she couldn't have any since she had to eat everything without salt. Someone whispered something to the waitress, and in a few minutes, she returned from the kitchen. Audrey smiled. It was a special plate of French fries without salt.

They had decided to spend the night in prayer at the grotto. The shifts were distributed while the dinner plates were cleared. Everyone was tired, but they had come for this purpose. It would be uncomfortable, in the empty enclosure, with a damp cold that chilled to the bone. It was drizzling outside. The gate near the grotto was closed, so they would have to go around the long way, one by one. It would be a prayer of resistance, of few words and much littleness. Much trust. Much faith.

The next morning, they had Mass at Vert Couret, a dairy farm about six miles from the Grotto of Lourdes which served as a center of reflection and study. It was there that Father Pierre, Omer, and Caroline had first received the news of Audrey's illness. Lillian remembered that the last time she had been in Lourdes was to attend a convention in 1989. Before leaving Paris, Audrey had said, "Mummy, when you're in Lourdes, will you go to the chapel where I made my first holy Communion?" She strongly insisted, making her mother understand the importance of her petition.

"Fine, Audrey, I'll do what I can."

Deep down, she didn't have any great desire to fulfill this wish. On one of the days of the convention, all the ladies went from Vert Couret down to the grotto to pray and go to the baths. Lillian recalled: "Audrey, ah, the chapel of her first holy Communion...." She didn't really remember where it was, and she wasn't looking forward to walking all over by herself to find it. In the end, she did set out looking for it, but only because Audrey had asked her. She entered the crypt. "Which was the chapel?" They were all the same. A rope blocked off the passageway, but she slipped under it. There was no one around, not even the Blessed Sacrament. Dull. Empty. Alone. She stood in front of a little altar to see if she had come upon the place. There, something happened. Lillian received a grace from the Lord that totally changed her life, her understanding of the faith, and her relationship with him. She came out transformed and deeply thankful to her daughter, asking herself if she would have received "that" if Audrey hadn't asked her to go.

After Mass, everyone got ready to go down to the baths at the grotto. Each one, in his heart, was offering this act for Audrey. Consciously or not, they took it as the last opportunity for...a miracle? Only God knew. He was the Lord. Lillian entered the baths with Audrey. There were some special ones reserved for sick people only. She prepared her. Luckily, there were few people around. It was quieter than usual. In that atmosphere, everything had the flavor of a prayer: the gestures, the movements, the glances.

"We are going to pray to Mary. We are going to put in her hands the intention we carry in the depths of our hearts. And," she added timidly, "we are also going to pray for you to be cured."

Audrey's gaze met her mother's eyes straight on:

"Mummy, I already know what I'm going to offer my bath for. It's for a young man who is doubting his vocation."

Just a few days ago, one of the Pink Ladies who had come to entertain her in the hospital in Paris had told her about the young man. He was hesitating about entering the seminary. After the bath, they were reunited with the others, and Jerome pushed Audrey's wheelchair. In the midst of overflowing joy, he carried a question nailed to his soul. He thought of Abraham, and it seemed to him that he was bringing his daughter to the altar of sacrifice like the patriarch had once brought Isaac. There were tears inside. "Do you not wish, Lord, to stay your arm?"

Such short and intense days. The conversations were simple; there was an eloquence about so much tenderness together. Everyone was praying to Mary, filled with the sense of her presence in the uncanny silence and atmosphere that one breathes in the air around the Grotto of Massabielle. They prayed for her intercession, asking for an end to Audrey's suffering, asking for her to stay with them. They cried. And after crying, they laughed.

They lived extraordinary moments with Audrey beside them and in their hearts. The airplane touched down at Orly Airport. Jerome and Lillian had talked during the flight.

"Audrey," said Papa, "what do you think about going to Rome?"

"Oh, yes. Very good!"

"Great. That is, only if you're not too tired. Maybe you'd prefer that we go back home."

Audrey listened and thought. Papa kept inviting her. He hesitated before saying, "Maybe we could even have a private Mass with the Holy Father."

Audrey smiled and declared, with resolve and conviction, that she had always dreamed of going to Rome because for some time now she had wanted to visit St. Peter and St. Paul's prison.

in st. peter's prison

Who had told this little girl that such a place existed? Neither Lillian nor Jerome was exactly sure.

They departed for Rome without even going back home. Jerome, Lillian, Aline, McLean, and Audrey were all together, jumping from one city to another with great speed. Lillian remembered her first trip to Rome with the children in 1986. It was by car, from Paris. During the car ride, which was very long, Audrey asked her to tell the story of Our Lady of Guadalupe at least ten times. And the story of St. Elizabeth of Hungary, who shared her riches with the poor. Such memories! Papa called the Legionaries of Christ first to ask about lodging, and they gave him the address of a *pensione* run by nuns on the Via Aurelia Antica. He also spoke with his friend Aloïs, the Swiss Guard.

"We could be there in a few hours. Do you think it would be possible for us to have Mass with the Holy Father?"

"Jerome, my friend…I am not allowed to say, the decision is only made the night before."

"Well then, friend to friend, would you like me to come to Rome?"

The colonel got the point and laughing, answered, "I'd love to see you again. Come to Rome, and I'll call you this evening."

Upon arriving at the Fiumicino Airport, they rented a van so that everyone and the wheelchair could travel with them. They got onto the Raccordo Anulare, the main highway in Rome. Exit

1: Via Aurelia. From there, two exhausting hours searching for the nuns' *pensione*, which they neither saw nor found. Jerome felt exasperated by the narrow, crowded, and consummately disorderly streets of the Eternal City. Meanwhile, Audrey sat quietly in the back, praying her rosary. Jerome's internal temperature was getting hotter and hotter; Audrey kept praying the rosary. Finally, Papa said, "Nothing. It's clear that God doesn't want us to find these nuns. So, too bad for them—we'll go to another place."

They had passed by a bright and attractive Holiday Inn about six times, so he drove them straight to it, absolutely convinced that God wanted them to stay precisely there, end of discussion.

Jerome thanked God for having allowed mankind to invent the credit card. He didn't even have one lira on him. After such an intricate and involved adventure, what a relief to be able to hand over the Visa card and *voila!* everything was arranged.

"Yes," he commented to Lillian, "and on the return flight we'll figure out how to pay this fortune."

The next day, May 19, was Pentecost Sunday. There was a particular joy hidden behind Audrey's smile: they were all going to the house of the Legionaries, to the Center for Higher Studies of the priests and brothers. Years before, she had been to another center, the one on Aurelia Nuova. She remembered it well: after the dinner, the Legionary choir sang for them with their small band. She couldn't take her eyes off the drums. With a gesture, Father Gonzalo had invited her to come up front. Without even a shadow of embarrassment, she made for the drums. The Legionaries played a little music to "accompany" her and Audrey played the most deafening piece the seminary had ever heard. The dining room was full of laughter and smiles, and there was an air of victory in Audrey's eyes. Her cheeks were pink with pleasure, and she was so satisfied to have been able to make "a bit of noise."

Upon their arrival at the Center for Higher Studies, Brother Raymundo helped Jerome to get the wheelchair out of the car.

The young seminarian noticed that the wheelchair was too big for Audrey and that her feet could not be supported, which was unnecessarily uncomfortable and tiring for her. Nobody else had noticed and, naturally, Audrey hadn't mentioned it. He briskly found two young brothers with an enormous toolbox. They knelt down beside her and adjusted the chair to perfection. What kindness! Charity put into action, thought Lillian. Another brother held open the door to the chapel for Audrey, and her heavenly smile as she wheeled past him would remain engraved on his memory forever. After Mass, he mentioned her smile to all his companions, and months later he told Lillian that he would never forget the way that little girl thanked him.

The main celebrant of the Mass was Father Marcial Maciel, the founder and then general director of the Legionaries of Christ. Afterwards, the family waited for him outside, since he was planning to greet them. He arrived and bent down to give Audrey a kiss, and they received his founder's blessing. It had been no small encouragement to him to know that this little girl's suffering had been bearing so many fruits, supporting so many of the vocations of his spiritual sons and giving strength to the ones who would soon be coming along.

Now the expedition began. Mick's good luck! Audrey explained that she had "always" wanted to see the prison of St. Peter and St. Paul. And so, off they all went. They had all eaten early. There, in the midday sunshine, they carried the wheelchair up the stairs of the Plaza del Capitolio, the most important of the seven Roman hills. At their feet was the Roman Forum and St. Peter's prison was right next to the Curia. From the Capitolio, they went down some steep, old stairs, taking small and careful steps, until they reached a tiny door. The guard followed them with his eyes as Jerome and McLean carried the wheelchair down the stairs and Lillian carried Audrey in her arms. She was somewhat heavy for her mother's small frame, but she always wanted Mummy to carry her. Only in her arms did she feel less pain—the others didn't know how to do it as gently. Lillian smiled at her daughter's little whim. In reality, she suspected that she just wanted to be close to Mummy. Aline went down the stairs in little hops, carrying the bag full of medicines, looking here and there.

"Ma questi: cosa fanno?"[4] The guard thought that these "francesi" were either all completely crazy or that they had a particular devotion to that obscure hideaway. From the door, one couldn't see much. It felt humid, and it was dark. The jail was below ground level, accessible with difficulty even for able-bodied tourists. But Audrey wanted to go all the way down.

"If we've already come this far, well, let's go."

McLean took it with good humor. They crossed the narrow galleries by the light of small candles. The walls glistened with moisture, and they could see some fragments of Latin inscriptions on a marble block that had once been white. They arrived at a small enclosure where an altar had been placed. A thin stream of water trickled by. Was that all? That was all.

For Audrey, it was enough. Rome was not a museum, but a living sanctuary. The stones spoke. The floor taught. The air inspired prayers. Audrey thought: *Peter was here. Paul was here.* She had been deeply impressed by how this great apostle had managed to convert the jail guards who were keeping watch over him. He had baptized them right there, with the water that ran through the insalubrious spot. She thought about the hospital, her nurses, her doctors....

There, in that prison, she felt a mysterious and real blood coursing through her veins, much more real than her own tortured blood. It was the blood of the martyrs, shed for love of Christ. Now she understood that she was a little martyr as well. She had come to Rome without fear, to continue pouring herself out, drop by drop, dreaming of receiving the palm one day. She

---

4 "What are those people doing?"

would be a white martyr; she would be part of that multitude of those who have come out of the great tribulation, who have washed their robes and made them white in the blood of the Lamb.

Upon leaving, they spent some time exploring the edge of the Forum while Jerome went to get the car. There were the dirt paths, the flagstones worn down by the passing of centuries, the grass and the pieces of columns, friezes, lintels, and statues. Some gypsies were wandering about as well. One had to be careful, because they had mastered the art of robbing tourists. Jerome saw his family from the distance and waved. In his mind, the question struck: "Will Aloïs call about the Mass with the Pope?" During dinner, they were tired, nervous, and full of expectation. Nobody had called. Finally, at ten o'clock, Aloïs called.

"You can come, but no more than four people. I'll meet you at six in the morning at the door of Saint Anne."

Jerome turned to his family with joy in his eyes:

"That's it! We have the Mass with the Pope!"

However, their joy soon paled when they encountered a small problem: there were five of them. Jerome quickly concluded that McLean would not go to the Mass. But before he could say it, a discussion broke out between the girls.

"Audrey said she wants to stay, and she wants Mick to go!"

Then Aline insisted on staying so that Audrey and Mick could both go. For Audrey, it was extremely important that her Uncle McLean should see the Pope. She was sure that that would make him decide about his vocation to the priesthood. She had prayed unceasingly for that intention, and here was her golden opportunity. She couldn't let him escape! She stuck to her idea with an obstinacy and a fire that surprised her sister, who had very rarely seen Audrey like that before. Nevertheless, she fought for her point of view with decision.

Jerome had to intervene. He was aware that he had never before given a flat "no" to his daughter. Never had he given her a prohibition or an order. This time, he ordered with unmovable firmness.

"Audrey, it is decided, and it will be done as I have said. Mick stays, and you come to Mass."

Audrey protested.

"Audrey! I know you don't understand, but you have to obey. Sometimes it's that way. I'm asking you to obey even though right now you don't want to and you don't understand. Afterwards, if God wants it, you will understand."

Audrey listened with her eyes downcast, holding back her disgust. It was costing her deeply to renounce her desire. But her mind was made up, and she wasn't going to give in and agree unless Aline promised to ask the Holy Father to pray for Mick, so that he would find his vocation. She expressly wanted to give this role to her sister. That way, Aline would have something to say to the Holy Father.

Since it was already late, they didn't sleep for long. At a very early hour, they got ready to go. There were few words. Lillian dressed Audrey. Aline got dressed by herself without saying anything. There were so many thoughts inside. Mick was going too, for the ride. There was silence; the tension of the evening before had had an effect. In a little while, they would be with the Holy Father, the Vicar of Christ on earth.

The streets of Rome were still empty, and the day began slowly, with the slightest hint of light between the brown and gray rooftops. It was cool outside. At the entrance to St. Anne's, two Swiss Guards kept watch, wearing their gray and blue uniforms and navy blue berets. One of them stepped up to them in a gentlemanly way to ask them what they wanted, and they saw the smiling face of Colonel Aloïs. He signaled to his companion, and they entered.

After parking the car in a small patio next to the St. Damascus courtyard, they settled Audrey into her wheelchair. Two doves were pecking at the dark paving stones. Aline walked timidly with tears in her eyes from the cold. Jerome made a funny comment. Audrey looked all around. It already smelled like coffee. The elevator stopped on the second floor, and the Swiss Guards helped with Audrey's wheelchair. Monsignor Stanislaw received them in the library and commented to the other priests in a discreet tone:

"Yes, I know, she is dying. The Swiss Guard told me."

During Mass, Jerome observed that four nuns had taken seats on some chairs outside the chapel. He realized: *These Polish sisters, who take care of the Pope, have given up their seats so that we could come.* He couldn't communicate with them, but he looked at them with sweetness, as if to say, "Thank you for your kindness. You don't know what this means to us."

In return, some eyes spoke with even more sweetness: "May God bless you. We are praying with you for your daughter."

In Jesus' Arms

At the end of Mass, they were ushered into the library again and waited their turn. Behind them were many volumes in Spanish and a modern sculpture in bronze, one of those that Paul VI liked so much.

They were the last ones. The Pope drew near and greeted them. Jerome explained to the Holy Father that they were French and that they belonged to Regnum Christi. He presented Lillian, Aline, and Audrey. The Pope understood and said in French, "We will pray together." Jerome explained Audrey's state of health, and the Holy Father repeated several times in his characteristic accent, "Audrey, Audrey."

Audrey kept looking at Mummy; she wanted to say something to the Pope. Lillian spoke up. "Your Holiness, my daughter has something she would like to tell you."

The Holy Father came closer to Audrey, and she raised herself up out of the wheelchair. She was there in front, so small, with her swollen face and her red handkerchief on her head. The Holy Father bent down until his face was touching hers. She had such a soft voice. He wanted to hear her well. He encircled her with his arm. Audrey's tone of voice was high and thin, and she had difficulty speaking. Aline observed how her sister's lips were moving. The Holy Father was nodding his head. He looked into her eyes and responded; it was a true dialogue. How long did it last? One minute, three minutes…. No one ever knew what Audrey confided to the Holy Father. No doubt he sensed the powerful and secret action of the Holy Spirit in this girl, chosen by Christ to pour out graces of conversion and surrender upon so many souls.

Afterwards, the Holy Father greeted Aline. She said nothing. Audrey fixed her eyes on her sister as if to say, "What! You're not speaking? Tell him, Aline! I can't believe you're not going to tell him."

She had forgotten.

"Aline forgot to tell the Pope to pray for you," explained Audrey to her uncle when they met him outside. "But don't worry, because at that moment I asked Jesus to tell the Holy Father to pray for you."

The return flight to Paris—there was a great weight of impressions, emotions, and fatigue; what they had lived had far surpassed their expectations. The eruption of Mystery in their souls had hit them like a great wave breaking against a cliff. As the plane prepared to land at the Paris airport, Lillian turned to her daughter.

"It's amazing, Audrey! Mother Teresa has held you in her arms, Father Maciel, LC, too, and now the Pope! What more could you want?"

Immediately, the little girl gently whispered: "For Jesus to hold me in his arms."

sign of contradiction

The families that gathered for the Tuesday Rosary thought that they were going to help Audrey, but it was Audrey who helped them through their own prayers. By praying, they meant to lead Audrey to health, but it was she who led them to health.

Up to that moment, many people had prayed for Audrey with an unaccustomed fervor. One has to understand the atmosphere that was created around her; it was much more than her parents had realized in the first days. Adults and children in Versailles kept praying for her every Tuesday at 8:00. The children of the Theresian mission kept praying for her with Father Thévenin.

And for many, the photograph of Audrey was already something to cherish and keep. One lawyer kept it in his briefcase. A journalist kept it in his agenda. A doctor had it close to him, on his desk. A seminarian looked at it before closing his prayer book. A priest used it to mark the day in his breviary. Audrey's photo. Besides that, there were all those other people, like those fathers of families who had never prayed in their lives and were now on their knees to save a little girl. They were starting to like this experience of going down on their knees, and prayer was starting to fill them.

But Audrey wasn't getting better. What was happening? They all thought they were helping Audrey with their prayers. They were convinced that God would come down from heaven to cure her. Perhaps they had been mistaken. Now, Audrey was clever; she knew that those prayers were actually helping them to recover their health. Her little fingers had opened the locked gates so that, with every Hail Mary they prayed for her, they would receive into their souls a little bit of heaven, a little bit of God, a little bit of the divine life that helps to heal and cleanse the deep wounds of our existence and illuminate the dark corners. They didn't know this, but they had never let go of Audrey.

When they heard that the transplant had failed, they were all frightened. They had spent months praying the Rosary every Tuesday; it was already part of their lives, and they had learned so many things. From her hospital bed, Audrey was the heart of this new family, an outlet of divine blood, the yeast in the dough, the source of unity and hope. What would happen to them without her? Would the Blessed Virgin also abandon them? How would they feel that sense of spiritual strength, the warmth of their common prayer? Would this special visit of heaven that had renewed the hearts of children and adults alike be ended in one stroke? They had been improving in their families and had just learned to pray. Would they be able to keep going without her help? Jerome and Lillian discovered that there was much more terror in the eyes of their friends than in their own. They were fortunate in that they felt led by the hand of the Lord. Nevertheless, how would they explain to all these children that their prayers, their sacrifices, and their efforts had been useless? It would cause a sense of disillusionment.

Upon their return from Rome, Jerome had decided that they would make no more trips to pray for the cure of their daughter. Now the telephone calls came pouring in.

"Listen, if you bring your daughter to Medjugorje, she'll be cured for sure."

They were from unknown people of all sorts.

"I know a healer in the south of France, and I'm sure he could do something for your daughter."

They were offered paramedical treatments, miraculous cures, magic—a veritable avalanche of human wills bent on the cure of Audrey. They also sought out Lillian, giving her bits of cotton soaked in healing oil. She received handkerchiefs bathed in the tears of some visionary, relics for her daughter to touch.... An interior instinct of modesty, respect, and reverence towards God led them to set all of these aside. He had accompanied them up to that moment, and he was wisely guiding the unfolding of his plans for his daughter. They had now set up a paradoxical barrier: they would not insist on the topic. They gave their full assent to the Lord's will and his plan for Audrey. God was God.

CHAPTER 5

BETWEEN HEAVEN AND EARTH

"Jesus and his Mother frequently chose children in order to entrust to them works of great importance for the life of the Church and of humanity.... It seems that the Redeemer of man shares with them his care for others.... He always listens to their prayers. What enormous strength has the prayer of a child!"

LETTER OF POPE JOHN PAUL II TO CHILDREN

Last Treatment

The month of May was almost over. *On prend un jour à la fois.* This meant living in the present, taking one day at a time. Once it was decided that Audrey would live at home, the doctors gave precise directions about the conditions for hygiene and immunity that had to be met in the room where she would sleep. Everything had to be impeccable, disinfected, new, and washable.

Audrey's room was up the stairs on the left, the only room with a balcony opening out onto the front garden and the quiet street. The bed was facing the window. From there, one could see the swaying branches of an enormous cherry tree, which cast an interplay of light and shadow in the afternoons. They tore down the old, dirty wallpaper, which was a dreadful orange color. They had to find something new. Lillian went with Audrey to choose the sample. There was a pale green pastel color that was transparent, gentle, and luminous. It would go well. But they had to choose some kind of decoration for the border.

"How about that one with the wildflowers?"

"No, Mummy, this one."

"This one?"

"Yes, Mummy, the one with the ducks."

It was decided, and that was the end of the discussion. At home, Audrey lay down, smiling, her face snuggled in the pillow. Playful and satisfied, her eyes followed a line of yellow ducks that marched proudly along the border in procession, and she greeted them from below.

Now they were going to give her an experimental chemotherapy treatment, the last chance. Various people had counseled them against it, saying that it would be of no use. Nevertheless, it was difficult to say no to a possible cure, even though the chances were at most minimal. They arrived at the hospital in the morning, and Mick was with them. He had wanted to come to play with Audrey and keep her company. Audrey climbed onto the bed. It was too high for her, and it was hard for her to climb onto it. She got settled and arranged the sheets while commenting in English: "Really, Mick, spending a day in the hospital isn't going to be very fun for you."

Even now, in the last phase of her illness, she wasn't thinking of herself. Even now, before her last treatment, which was to see if they could extend her life a little bit, she was more worried that her uncle Mick would be bored during a day in the hospital.

Lillian suffered, thinking about the days that had to follow. How would she prepare her daughter for death? Doctors and family members that were advising Jerome and Lillian insisted that Audrey should be told she was soon going to die. Lillian thought to herself: *How do you tell your eight-year-old child she is going to die? And what if, after all, a miracle was still possible...?* Audrey was very close to her mother. If she even thought of the day of her death, wouldn't she mostly be afraid to be separated from her?

Finally, Lillian got up the courage to say: "You know, Audrey, that if a day comes when you have to go to heaven before me, I am sure that you will find your true mother there. She will take very good care of you—you'll see—because she loves you much more than I ever could."

Audrey looked at Lillian.

"Ah, yes! I know that very well."

Her eyes shone with joy. Lillian realized the absurdity and the uselessness of her worries. Audrey was waiting for heaven with all her heart.

Audrey at Home, and Jesus too

Mummy prepared the children: "We have to be very careful with Audrey, and you have to be very clean in order to be with her. Don't get too close to her. Don't bring dirt into the house or leave anything dirty near her. If you go into her room, don't touch the doorknob with your hands. Open it with your elbow so that you don't leave germs."

The children, impressed, followed these instructions to the letter. Aline went into Audrey's room, noticing that it was not easy to open the door. What to do? Why with the elbow? When she came in, Audrey looked at her. "Mummy told you to open it like that, right?"

Aline sat down, and with a smile said, "Sorry, I couldn't do anything else."

Beatrice, so tiny, held Grégoire's hand and attempted a genuflection. She was two years and four months old.

Now, Jesus had come to live with them at home. Yes, he lived in that special box that was in the chapel of their house. The privilege of having Audrey with them had brought with it the privilege of having the Blessed Sacrament in their home! The bishop had agreed; it was only for a while.... They had asked permission through the parish priest of La Celle St. Cloud. Much later, Jerome had the opportunity to greet the bishop.

He said, "Your Excellency, I am the father of the girl who had leukemia. You gave us permission to have the Blessed Sacrament in our house."

The bishop remembered the petition perfectly.

With Audrey, only marvelous things happened. The chapel became the family's favorite place to be. Audrey spent hours there in silence, her eyes fixed on the simple tabernacle. The little room was filled with sunlight, with its white rays in the clarity of the morning and its warm, velvet caress in the late afternoon. A gentle breeze carried in the spring fragrance of the garden.

People came to visit them. They came to see Audrey. The house in La Celle St Cloud had changed. In the midst of the natural joy and noisiness of the children, there was a certain new air of peaceful recollection.

"Come on in. In a moment you will see Audrey. She's in

the chapel." They opened the door halfway. Audrey didn't turn around to look. Whoever entered didn't dare to interrupt her— she was so recollected! They remembered with embarrassment and discomfort how much noise they had made with their greetings upon entering the house. Upon leaving, they instinctively resumed their conversation in a low voice. Granny spent some days at home with them. She loved to stay in prayer with her granddaughter and observe her. She was her living sermon.

The door to the chapel opened slowly and awkwardly. It was Beatrice; she had pushed it open with her little body, almost losing her balance because in her hands she was carrying a juicy apple. It seemed like she was coming forward with great satisfaction to offer the apple to her big sister. But oh! Audrey looked right at her and said with gentleness and firmness, "Beatrice, no. Not in here with the apple. Take it out."

Startled, without saying a word, Beatrice immediately turned around and went out with a solemn air. Right away, she entered again, brushing off her hands. The apple was gone. Her blue eyes turned to Audrey, seeking a look of approval. She put her hands on Audrey's knees and smiled. Audrey smiled in return. Granny smiled, too, impressed. "My granddaughter has real authority."

confirmation, american style

Granny had asked Audrey, "What do you do when you wake up in the morning?"

She answered, "I pray, and I wait."

Audrey was a girl, a little virgin on foot with her lamp burning, waiting for the arrival of her Spouse. Her sickness had forged her capacity to wait. Her body had learned to wait. Her mind had learned to wait. Her emotions waited. She waited in suffering, holding on for a minute of relief in the midst of pain. It was the waiting of her soul. She waited, sitting in her bed, for the nurse to come and open the curtains. She waited quietly, tied down, while the machines probed her body. She waited for Mummy's arrival. She waited with fear for the moment of the spinal tap. She waited with joy for the coming of a priest. She waited to go home. She waited to reunite herself with Jesus in the Eucharist. She waited for the decision of her Uncle Mick, counting bead after bead on her rosary. She waited to touch the hand of Mummy after coming out of the sterile bubble. She waited for Jesus to embrace her. She waited for heaven.

Her soul was ready to receive a gift from on high. "Come, Holy Spirit." Mummy and Papa arranged everything with the parish priest. Audrey would soon receive the sacrament of confirmation. Lillian looked for a booklet to prepare her; she doubted whether she would know how to explain the meaning of the sacrament, the gifts of the Holy Spirit.... She eyed the pages and searched her memory; there were things that even she didn't understand well, and her catechism lessons seemed very distant. She sat down next to her daughter and they talked. Less than ten minutes went by, and Lillian was overjoyed and surprised. Audrey's soul already possessed everything that was necessary to know in order to receive the sacrament. She even understood much better than her mother.

Lillian realized that Audrey had no one to teach her. Audrey, totally open and penetrated by prayer, was a log in the fire of the Holy Spirit that had been consuming itself for some time. The damp log had already stopped smoking. The black firebrand had already changed. It had already turned from black to white ash, and from white to red, like the red fire.

Audrey, full of enthusiasm, prepared everything with Mummy. It had to be a big party, a real fête. She chose the hymns, and she named Omer to read one of the readings, which she herself had chosen. Lillian, who knew how precise her daughter's ideas were, brought her to the supermarket to choose the pastries for the party. And did she ever have precise ideas! They had to buy the best, or rather, the most chocolaty. And not only that—she spent hours placing the pastries on six trays. Mick watched her, marveling at her perfectionism. Mummy brought out all the pretty things of the house: the silver trays, the lace tablecloths.... Audrey also chose holy cards to commemorate the day, painstakingly writing the date and her name on each one. They were placed on a wooden tray that she had decorated with McLean by gluing on a whole series of photographs of animals and then varnishing it.

On June 1st, Audrey received the sacrament of confirmation in her house. A parish priest came, sent by the bishop, and the whole family made an effort to be there, as well as their closest friends. Brigitte was once again Audrey's godmother, and after the ceremony, Father Thévenin stopped by to see them. Audrey was happy. That day, they had done things as well as possible. God, too. With his Spirit, he had renewed the face of the earth.

châteauneuf de galaure

Jerome and Lillian had said that they were finished with trips and pilgrimages after Rome. That was enough trotting from here to there. They had Jesus at home; what more could they want?

This time, though, it was Brigitte. She lived with her husband and children in Grenoble, and she was very involved with a spiritual foyer in Châteuneuf de Galaure. There, a woman named Marthe Robin had lived and died. Sick from childhood, she had spent years without leaving her bed. On her bed of pain, each week she experienced the sufferings of the passion of our Lord. Brigitte was very devoted to this mystic and had heard that a miracle was necessary in order to accelerate the process of her beatification. Maybe if Audrey went and prayed in her room and was healed.... Brigitte asked them to come; she insisted, but to no avail. She told them the priest in charge of the foyer wanted them to come. Finally, they decided to go, not for a cure but to please Brigitte, such a loving godmother. Besides, Audrey would see her cousins. She got ready for the trip. They were going to stay in a retirement home in Châteauneuf that was run by some consecrated lay women. Audrey, with her usual wry sense of humor, warned Aline, "You'll see—they'll give us soup." And of course they did!

Audrey loved her godmother very much and fell in love with Châteauneuf de Galaure. The fields of high Provence were filled with the fragrance of wheat and hay, with a tapestry of bluebells, poppies, and violets everywhere. They could already see Marthe Robin's house. Here the sky was enormous. When you looked far off, the furrows joined the sky. Far away, an almond tree, an apple tree, and a walnut tree dotted the golden earth. They arrived at the house, which was a sandy color and bathed in sunshine. The sloped roof was made of Mediterranean tile. Lilies and rosebushes stirred in the breeze. A cat and a puppy were there, too. To the east, shadowed fields; to the west, sun-soaked fields. To the north, the fields stretched into infinity. And to the south, the fields extended to satiety.

Marthe's room was small and dark, full of furniture, framed memorabilia, and old photos. Upon entering, one saw the mystic's bed to the right. Behind her bed was the window, which was mostly closed during her life, since the light hurt her eyes. The rickety bed was nailed to the wall, which was lined with wood from the floor to about a meter and a half in height. The bedspread was white, with old-fashioned lace. The room gave one a sudden shock upon entering. Audrey had gone on ahead. Lillian drew near to the door and listened from the threshold.

"Come see, Mummy. Marthe's room is impressive. More impressive than seeing the Pope."

Lillian, in silence and praying within, began to cry. Audrey took her by the hand. "Mummy, it's as if we were in heaven."

In the retirement home, there were old nurses among the residents, some of whom were in wheelchairs. What jolly merrymaking in the dining room! That was worth seeing. Audrey was happy to be able to share her salt-free food with them. Mummy had found some especially good products in a shop in Versailles, and Audrey was delighted to share these rare delicacies. The old people looked at her, patted her hand, and tears leapt into their eyes when they heard her talk about her visit to Marthe Robin's room. Audrey continued talking and told them that she had just recently made her confirmation "American style." The old people, taken aback, repeated to each other what she had just said.

"In the United States, the children make their confirmation when they're young, together with the profession of faith. In France, it is done separately," she explained.

Many did not manage to understand it, but it amused them, and they talked about it, smiling and looking at her. A *l'américaine!* Audrey explained it again, as many times as they asked her. She was pleased to have awakened so much interest in these older people.

During those days, everyone was hanging on the results of the blood tests. Brigitte made frequent telephone calls. There was no change, and they understood that God's ways were not their ways.

Intimacy with Jesus

June was a pleasant and happy month. The house felt full with Audrey home, and Mrs. Barbé came to sit with her to teach her new things.

Audrey continued with her interest in the game called The Promised Land, a game that demanded great doses of patience. It consisted of a desert drawn on a board, with some wandering figures that had to cross it in order to reach the Promised Land. Each player moved forward if he could successfully answer a question chosen by his adversary. The questions were all based on more or less obscure details from the Bible. It took hours to find the answers to the game's questions, and once you found them, bang!

A trap! Then, when you were just about to reach the end, you'd get one of those deadly questions that sent you right back to the beginning again.

Audrey loved to put the priests who came to visit her into a tight spot with that game, especially Father Pierre and Father Thévenin. She would look for an especially difficult question, and then would ask it with mischievous delight, carefully guarding the answer. She also played word games; there was one game in which she had made herself a specialist in the hospital. First, one had to choose a very big and difficult word from the dictionary. Then, one had to make a list of the words that could be made from the letters within it. The winner was the one who found the most words.

On St. Audrey's day, the 23rd of June, Father Thévenin came to celebrate Mass. Audrey prepared for the Mass with great care. For that day, she invented a singing response to the prayers of the faithful and chose her favorite psalm: "The Lord is my Shepherd."

The school year was coming to an end. Audrey saw her siblings come home happy; soon, they would all be on vacation. On some Saturdays, they went out to picnic in the gardens of the Versailles Palace. Audrey looked off into the distance. The Great Canal receded to a point with the two rows of black poplars that lined its banks. Beyond that, it was all woods and sky. Children chased each other among the hedges. There were tourists everywhere. A Japanese man was taking pictures of his children, who were so cute and joyful among the petunias, the begonias, and the chrysanthemums.

They returned to the peaceful silence of their home. The little chapel candle flickered; the Lord was here. Audrey entered, full of enthusiasm. Just to see her was enough to awaken a real curiosity: what would she and Jesus say to each other? This was Audrey's territory, her secret garden with the treasure of an intimate friendship.

One night Lillian closed the door to Audrey's room after her. Like all nights, Lillian had spent a long moment next to Audrey's bed, talking with her, saying her evening prayers, and then kissed her goodnight. She was about to go down the stairs but, on a sort of impulse, turned back, opened the door a crack, and looked out of the corner of her eye. She wanted to see her one more time. What a surprise! Audrey was kneeling on her bed with her face to the wall. It would have been exhausting for her to pull herself up into this position, she who couldn't even sit up in bed without help. She drew her face as close as she could to the image of Christ that hung over her bed and gave it a kiss. When she lay down again to sleep, mother and daughter's eyes met. Lillian closed the door, blushing a bit, like someone who had just invaded another's moment of intimacy. Audrey had smiled at her without saying a word.

school friends

On Saturday afternoon, the Capuchin priests of Versailles celebrated Mass for the end of the school year for the students of Les Châtaigniers. Audrey had a great desire to go. At the entrance to the church, she saw familiar faces; many had been meeting at the Tuesday Rosary. Audrey came into the church, Aline pushing her wheelchair, and there was a stir as all the children turned in their pews to see her. A little boy touched his mother's arm: "Maman, it's Audrey!"

Yes, he had never seen her before, but he had come a few times to the Tuesday Rosary, and he had her little card on his night table. The lady, impressed, followed Audrey with her gaze. Her face had been deformed by the treatments; she was wearing a bandana on her head and that angelic smile. Audrey waved. She was radiant. It had been a year since she had seen her school friends. They settled her in front to the left, and she followed the Mass in her missal. They saw her moving her lips, singing the responsorial psalm. It was her last appearance in public. Upon arriving home, they carried her up to her room. She was so happy, and once in bed, she told Lillian, "Mummy, today I saw all my friends!"

convulsions

It was Sunday. Audrey tried to get out of bed and fell. Lillian arrived quickly and saw her. She thought she had lost her balance. She picked her up carefully and put her back onto her bed. That night, the convulsions started. Lillian didn't leave her side for an instant. Audrey was rigid, her eyes turned back in her head; she would shake, stop for a moment, and then it would start again. She felt it coming. Lillian caressed her arm and her hands, speaking gently to her. Audrey couldn't speak and her eyes were closed, but Lillian felt that she could hear: "Mummy is here. Don't worry." It was important to be close to her. It was impossible to reach a single doctor. She didn't want to take Audrey to the emergency room. What was happening? What was going to happen next? Lillian prayed the Rosary for her, and ended up falling asleep at her side. Four hours, five hours went by....

The next morning, Audrey's hands were clenched. One hand jumped all the time, while she couldn't move the other. She wasn't able to focus or control her eyes. This meant that the sickness had attacked her central nervous system. She was also unable to speak for a while. From then on, she would gradually lose all her faculties and the control of her movements. Nevertheless, she was completely lucid until the end, and she took all these things with indefatigable humor. She was able to laugh at herself, like the time when her aunt Brigitte came to see her and she told her, "How funny! Look at my hand—it jumps like a frog." Audrey's next task was to regain the use of her hands, a task that took great effort and dedication. At the beginning, she wasn't even able to hold a pen, but with willpower, she was able to write again.

One of those days, they brought her to the hospital for a blood transfusion, and the professor came to visit her. Lillian had explained how this doctor, who was so important, had worried about her and how much he cared for her, but Audrey was not convinced. She thought that the professor didn't spend enough time with his patients, and that he barely knew them because he spent too much time in front of his computer and his files. The professor watched her as she wrote with difficulty and courage.

"Are you managing to write?"

Without saying anything, she held out the sheet of paper. The professor read, "Etienne" (Stephen). It was his name. He was very struck by this, because he didn't realize that Audrey knew his first name. The message was clear: "I know you, and you don't come often enough to see me."

At the beginning of July, they decided to organize all of Audrey's transfusions and medical care at home. No more exhausting, gloomy trips to the hospital. In the morning, some nurses came to give Audrey her injections, change the bandages on her catheter, and take blood samples. The doctor, Aimé, a friend of the family, visited them, and Uncle Marc kept in touch with Lillian by telephone. One day, somebody made a comment in Audrey's hearing about what became of the body after death. Appalled, Lillian took the first opportunity to whisper to Audrey: "Audrey, you know, that isn't—" She was cut off short. "Mummy, I know. The body is just like a dress: when it becomes too small, it is put away in the cupboard…."

Messages for Heaven

They thought that Audrey would die very quickly. She could no longer move, and she could hardly eat. Her state of fatigue was intense. An avalanche of people came to entrust their prayer intentions to her— she was so close to heaven! At home, the doorbell was constantly ringing, and up to ten people visited in one day, asking for all sorts of things. They all came with all their intentions. Behind those faces and worries, there were people who couldn't hide an undefined spiritual restlessness. There were some who came with a good dose of curiosity. There were some who wanted to come and accompany and console a sick girl. For Lillian, it was difficult to know how to manage the situation.

"Mummy, why did this lady 'divide from' her husband?" (That's what Audrey called divorce.)

Audrey took things so much to heart that she really suffered for the intentions entrusted to her. This exhausted her even more. Nevertheless, Lillian knew how powerful Audrey was in prayer, and she couldn't close the door on them. They all left profoundly moved. There was something about Audrey that didn't leave them the same. Jerome had a cousin who was an Orthodox priest. He lived nearby, so they called him on the phone asking that he come to see Audrey, and he spoke with her for just a few minutes. After his visit, he admitted that he was very moved. "I thought that I came to bring something to Audrey, but it was actually she who gave me everything."

Father Pierre came often during those days and spent long periods of time with Audrey. He spoke to her, prayed with her, and put his apostolic projects in her hands. One afternoon, he took Aline and Henry aside and explained to them in a very kind and simple way that Audrey would soon be going to heaven. From there, she would continue her mission. He knew, deep down, that beyond his own words, it would be Jesus the Master who would prepare them for that moment.

Audrey took the intentions entrusted to her very seriously. She asked Lillian to keep track of them in a notebook, but one day she told her, "They have asked me to pray for so many things! Do you think I could tell Jesus that I'm praying for all that they have entrusted to me without repeating the intentions one by one?" Lillian, a little impatient that people would burden a sick child with their own preoccupations, readily said, "Yes." Yes, of course—the Lord already knew the intentions. Audrey tried it like that for two days, although she soon changed her mind.

"No, Mummy, this isn't good. I should pray for each intention."

She put Lillian in charge of writing down and reading each one, but she perfectly remembered each thing that they had asked her, as well as who had asked it. When she prayed, she formulated the precise intention and the name of the person who had asked it. Even though Lillian insisted that it wasn't necessary to repeat each thing, Audrey continued to name them separately. For God, every soul was important—every suffering, every prayer.

we are going to Normandy

Paris began to empty out now that summer vacation time had arrived and it was getting hot. The children were dreaming of the pool, of the sea. Audrey was very sick…nevertheless, life went on. "The others" packed their suitcases and went to the country-side, to the mountains, to the sea. Audrey's grandparents, uncles, and cousins were settled at Maillot. Audrey remembered too: the farm, the pool, the cherry tree…. Lillian and Audrey stayed in Paris alone, waiting. After only a few days, Lillian decided to bring Audrey to the country. She didn't want to just wait. They organized everything, even though it was difficult to move all the medical equipment to Maillot and risky to have the transfusions there. If something happened, the closest hospital was an hour away in Caen. But in spite of everything, the little girl would be happy with the garden, the flowers, and the sky. They set out for Normandy, and Audrey was radiant. When they arrived at Maillot and took Audrey out of the car, she was smiling, so happy to see everyone again.

But as Lillian took her in her arms to bring her inside, Audrey burst into tears and cried disconsolately.

"What's wrong, Audrey? Aren't you happy we've come to Maillot?"

Between sobs, she responded, "Yes. But my Lord isn't here."

What disappointment! It was true; they hadn't been able to bring Jesus. He had stayed at home in his chapel with his red light and his tabernacle. He meant everything to her, and there was no way of taking this thorn from her side. When a neighboring priest, Father Jean Bernard, began to come to the house to celebrate Mass, Audrey would always ask him in her delicate voice, "Are you sure that we couldn't make a little chapel here? Can't you leave the Lord with us?"

Father, with sorrow and with tenderness, had to explain once again that he couldn't because he needed permission from the bishop.

sunflowers

Everyone received the news of Audrey's arrival at Maillot with great joy. Her grandparents and four of her aunts and uncles—Lillian's siblings—were there, including McLean and Rose. Audrey spent as much time with them as she was able. It was something new for her aunts and uncles to see such a small creature acting with the maturity and poise that she had acquired during her sickness and suffering. On more than a few occasions, she surprised them with her reactions. Audrey ate with everyone at the dining room table; actually, it was more to be with everyone than to eat, since she could barely swallow any food. This was indescribably hard for her. Sometimes she had to get up immediately to go to the bathroom because she could no longer control all of her bodily functions. Lillian helped her, supported her, or put her in the wheelchair.

In that house, they didn't say grace, but Audrey kept up her usual custom of saying grace before every meal. When seated next to her grandfather, she said it in English, just loud enough so that he could benefit by it. She said it under her breath, but nevertheless, the others noticed the way she recollected herself, how she joined her hands…. One day, having noticed the detail, and a little piqued, her uncle Alexander commented, "But Audrey, if we have to give thanks to God every time we eat, then we should be giving him thanks all the time, for everything!"

"Yes, that's right," replied Audrey, with a sweet, convinced smile.

One must mention that for the young American, it was an answer that would stay with him for the rest of his life.

Among other activities, they spent long periods of time in the "Blue Room." They put Audrey on a blue sofa by the door, propped up with cushions, so that everyone could see her, and so that she could participate in the life of the household. They talked and played cards, Monopoly, and The Promised Land. When they got together to have a snack, Uncle Mick lit a fire in the fireplace. He knew how much Audrey loved watching the bright flames dance in the hearth.

After dinner, everyone went out for a walk. Evenings in Normandy have a magic charm, and in the summer the sun sets late. It was a good time to enjoy the sunset. The house was surrounded by fields, and the children bicycled happily on the winding driveway, while others played with a ball. They brought Audrey along in a stroller, and they all enjoyed the smell of the wildflowers, the wheat fields, and the grass. The breeze surrounded them with its summery scent, and the sky was dyed with the most splendid colors and reflections, like a royal display of stained glass. It was neither the blazing sun of the Mediterranean nor the pallid light of the northern countryside. It was just right. One walked, quiet and thoughtful, bathed in the serene blue and peaceful light. It was impossible not to remember the laughter of the Little Prince in the field of gold. On one of those evenings, a spectacular sunset lit up the sky, and there were exclamations of admiration and joy.

"It looks like a painting!"

"Yes, almost like a watercolor! It's magnificent."

Several of them wanted to go running back to the house to fetch a camera. Lillian heard Audrey softly murmur, "Thank you, Jesus."

Games with Madame Barbé

During this period, Audrey had some moments of great vivacity. It wasn't necessary to "keep her company," since she had learned to keep herself entertained. In her room, she wrote and wrote: she wrote letters and secret codes for her brothers and sisters, she recopied her prayers and favorite songs, and she frequently read her book of Bible stories.

Lillian installed a baby monitor so that she could always hear what was going on in Audrey's room when she was downstairs. One day, when she was talking with the others in the living room, she overheard Audrey speaking to someone in a rather didactic tone. She went upstairs, and to her surprise, found Grégoire seated on Audrey's bed, very attentively receiving a serious catechism lesson from his sister.

Mrs. Barbé came to see her again; now they no longer studied, but they did play with spirit. The lady watched with great tenderness how Audrey staged a little play with her siblings and cousins. We can already imagine: she gave out the roles, explained the lines, and directed the rehearsal. Installed in a big yellow armchair, she was quite happily in charge.

Mrs. Barbé explained to Audrey that she would not be coming back soon. "You see, my mother is sick; she's a bit old, and I have to go take care of her."

"Well, yes, your mother must be old," answered Audrey, looking closely at the wrinkled face of the good lady. Mrs. Barbé couldn't help bursting into laughter.

Ten minutes from the house, good friends were also on their summer vacation: Odile, Geoffroy, and their children. One afternoon, Henry and Aline were playing at their friends' house when they found a baby hedgehog on the edge of a path. That was a real treasure. The children got to work: they had to pick it up and put it in a box without getting stuck by its spines. The operation was conducted in silence and with great concentration, while the other children watched and kept quiet. They brought it to Odile and Geoffroy's house and put it in the kitchen, poking their noses close to the box, wanting to see the little animal close up. There were excited squeals and exclamations when the little creature began to move, and when its paws scratched at the box, wanting to get out. The afternoon was spent in the most delightful way, with a thousand and one opinions and suggestions about what the hedgehog should eat, how it should be cared for, if its mother had left it behind…. Then they had an idea:

"Hey—why don't we bring it to Audrey for her to see?"

There was unanimous agreement, and the mascot was accompanied by a small crowd of young children. They were so excited that they almost crushed it on the way. When they arrived, everyone tiptoed in so as to surprise Audrey.

"Audrey, look—a present!"

Everyone came into the room. That was not a moment to be missed. Audrey sat up in her wheelchair. "What is it?"

They brought the box to her. The only sound was the breathing of the children. They wanted to see Audrey's face and they wanted to see the hedgehog. Audrey's face lit up with joy. What a nice hedgehog! They spent some time with her, and for Audrey, it was heaven: her best friends and her brothers and sisters were all around her, and this little creature, too. With great attention, she listened to the exciting story of how they had captured the hedgehog and managed to put it in the box amidst such arduous and painful difficulties. It was an extraordinary success for her to share in the midst of the monotony of waiting.

Father Jean Bernard

Today they were preparing the room in a special way. Father Jean Bernard, Geoffrey's brother, had arrived from Italy and was coming to celebrate the Mass. The month of August was beginning. Finally, they would see Jesus at home, and Audrey would receive him. McLean was to be the acolyte at Mass. Audrey had not stopped praying for him. Before starting the Mass, Audrey's gaze searched all around for Mummy. When she saw her, she was reassured. Mummy was very much in her prayers because Audrey knew that even though she was surrounded by the mystery, she was not always able to comprehend it. Before Father Jean Bernard left the house, Lillian discreetly mentioned something to him. The priest went to Audrey's room; she had asked for confession.

"Father, will you come tomorrow to celebrate Mass?"

"Not tomorrow, but the day after tomorrow, yes."

"And couldn't you leave Our Lord here in the house, just for a day?"

This happened frequently after Masses in the house during the first two weeks of August. Audrey had acquired the habit of asking the priest to hear her confession every day that he came. Lillian felt a bit uncomfortable.

"But Audrey, do you think it's necessary for you to have confession every day? Father is in a hurry; surely he has things he needs to do."

"Mummy, when one has been confirmed, one knows perfectly well what is good and what is bad."

Audrey said it with seriousness. She said it with respect. Once again, Audrey had spoken.

Some time later, Aline came back from her summer camp in Lourdes with a printed card that Audrey noticed. They were some simple prayer commitments that Aline had promised Jesus to do every day in order to be a better friend to him and to save souls.

Although Aline was younger than all the other girls in the camp, the counselors gave her permission to make her promise because she was so enthusiastic to do so. She told Audrey about it, who then added right away: "I want to do it too."

Father Jean Bernard was a bit surprised. In confession, Audrey carefully examined a sheet full of boxes marked with a little cross where she had noted down whether she had fulfilled her prayers well or not: the offering of her day, a mystery of the rosary, being good to her brothers and sisters, and being obedient to her mother and father.

"Yes, Audrey had a kind of rule or regimen of life. She was very concerned about making sure that she had done each thing well to please Jesus," the priest said some time later. He always remembered Audrey as a girl who was very attentive to everything that kept her in the presence of God. Her perfectionism did not come from scrupulousness. In fact, her day revolved around her prayer. In the mornings, after getting ready, she would spend a good hour in prayer. Above all, Audrey was seeking to be good for Jesus. She wanted to please him in the little things. In confession and in conversation with the priest, she never brought up her sufferings or the things that bothered her. Her attention was centered, polarized, on her relationship with Jesus. By now, her whole life was a prayer: a prayer of loving self-offering, a prayer of intimate companionship, a prayer of union with the One she knew loved her.

I Hear voices

In the depths of her heart, Lillian wondered, "How long is this going to last?" Audrey and all of them were suspended between heaven and earth. One night, during the weekend of August 10th, they were saying their prayers as a family. Audrey was in bed, surrounded by Aline, Henry, the little ones, Brigitte (who was spending a few days with them), Mick, Granny, and Lillian. Each one was saying his or her intentions. Audrey's turn arrived:

"For mothers who have lost a child, so that they will understand that that child of theirs is a small servant of Christ in heaven."

She didn't say it for herself. She said it for Lillian. One of her aunts had just lost a son. He would be a servant of Christ in heaven.

In reality, Audrey was already serving Jesus in heaven. Lillian sensed it more and more strongly as the days went by. It was true; they were living on borrowed time, as if they had a visitor from heaven in their home. In their conversations and soul-sharing, it could be felt that Audrey was no longer of this world. She continued singing her little songs, but now she lived them. She continued saying her simple prayers, but now they sounded even more vibrant, more real, as if she were touching heaven with the tips of her fingers. Faith was no longer an abyss, an ocean to cross. Faith was a tenuous veil, now almost imperceptible. There was Audrey, and so resplendent were the things of God that she could no longer turn her gaze away. With amazement, Lillian followed in the footsteps of her daughter, still unaccustomed to the mystery of it all. For example, Audrey had told her that she wanted to dress all in blue, because the Blessed Virgin wore blue.

From the beginning of the month, Lillian's motherly fears grew stronger. It was inexplicable. She now slept in Audrey's room. Each day, Audrey woke up before her and began to sing, to pray. One day, she waited until Lillian woke up to tell her, "Mummy, I've been hearing voices lately."

"Voices?"

"Yes, inside. I hear the voice of Jesus, and at the same time, another."

"And what do they tell you?"

"Things. But sometimes I don't know if they are good voices or bad voices. Then I get scared and I don't want to listen to them."

"Well, I don't know what to say, Audrey. Maybe you can ask Father Jean Bernard. But I think that if these voices are telling you good things, thoughts that bring you closer to Jesus and give you the desire to be good, then they come from God. But if they are thoughts that take away your peace, frighten you, and are bad, then they are from the devil."

Audrey was not worried about hearing or not hearing. What worried her was not hearing the voice of her Lord for a single moment.

Now Lillian was in Paris because Jerome was in the hospital

with a collapsed lung. Brigitte had come to stay with Audrey so Lillian could spend the day at her husband's side. The Feast of the Assumption, August 15th, was already drawing near. It was also the anniversary of Audrey's first holy Communion. She shared her excitement with Aunt Brigitte. How much she loved her! Now Brigitte, seated on her bed, told her the story of St. Maximilian Kolbe. It was the 14th of August.

"...and then one day, during prayer, God offered him two crowns: one red, for martyrdom, and one white, for purity. He chose both."

"How I understand...."

At St. Thérèse's House

In the morning of August 15th, Father Jean Bernard came to the house to celebrate a solemn Mass for them; it was the Feast of the Assumption, a well-loved feast that has always been celebrated in France. Later in the day, Brigitte had to take the train with her daughter Anne Sophie to return to Brittany, so they planned to leave from the Lisieux station. Lillian and Aline accompanied Brigitte and Anne Sophie to the train station in Lisieux. Audrey had insisted on making the trip for her sister St. Thérèse... and for Brigitte too. As they waved goodbye, there were tears in Brigitte's eyes. Something told her that she would not see her niece again.

Afterwards, Lillian and Aline took Audrey to the Carmelite convent. They prayed in the chapel, in that place Audrey loved so much, where God had one day planted the seed of her interior life. They stayed there only a little while, for a few brief minutes, but they were so intense, so full, that they have remained permanently engraved on their souls. They visited the gift and souvenir shop and looked around, but they didn't really have much of a desire to buy anything. Audrey chose a small picture. She looked at it closely: it was a photo of St. Thérèse, with her pretty face and her crown of flowers, on her deathbed. She read it. "Have you seen it, Mummy?" she said with her smile. And she read the words out loud, "I am not dying, but entering into life."

⚕

On the morning of August 16th, Audrey was still sleeping. The entire household, including Audrey, had been up early, but Audrey had gone back to sleep. Lillian came into her room to check on her. As her mother watched her, she awoke between dreams, asking, "And Mick? Where is Mick?"

"He has left to go the seminary," Lillian assured her.

It was true. That very morning, McLean had packed his bags and left for Rome. They had all said good-bye, including Audrey. He had made his decision to become a priest and had enrolled in Mater Ecclesiae, a seminary for diocesan priests directed by the Legionaries of Christ. But even though she had said good-bye to Mick that very morning, his niece could not manage to assimilate it. She had carried that intention so deeply in her heart that she even remembered it in her dreams.

"Ah…then, now I can rest," breathed Audrey.

My Brothers And Sisters

That weekend of August 17th and 18th, Audrey felt very tired. Lillian did too. Since the convulsions started, she had slept in her daughter's room in order to take care of her at night

The following day, Monday, Father Thévenin had proposed celebrating Mass in Honfleur. He was spending his vacation there at his mother's house. Honfleur is a quaint fishing town almost an hour's drive from Maillot. Jerome's family knew of the little church overlooking the sea as a sanctuary where Masses were always offered for the dead. Every year, they used to make a little pilgrimage there. It was always a pleasant outing, with a picnic and games on the beach. This time, Lillian was very reluctant to bring Audrey. Audrey was determined to go, in spite of her lack of strength, and Lillian finally decided to take her. As usual, Audrey wanted to read the reading at Mass. But this time, she wasn't able to reach the end of it; her voice broke off from fatigue so Lillian finished it for her. After the Mass was over, Audrey wanted to see Father Thévenin in order to ask him what was the best and most exact way to make the Sign of the Cross. They had been debating at home whether one should say "Holy Spirit" touching two different shoulders, or whether one should say "Holy Spirit" touching the left shoulder, and "Amen" touching the right shoulder. That's Audrey....

On Tuesday the 20th, they had an appointment at the hospital in Caen for a transfusion. But Lillian doubted that Audrey would make it to that day. For the moment, she thought it best to send Aline and Henry to stay with their uncle Patrick, Jerome's eldest brother.

He had a very beautiful property, horses and all, an hour from Maillot. On Sunday afternoon, Aline went up to Audrey's room to say good-bye before leaving. Lillian found her on the stairs and said, "Tell her everything you want to say."

Aline went up in peace. She didn't really think it would be the last time she would see her. Lillian had told them before that "if something happens" she would call them immediately. Aline walked into the room. She had just turned ten years old. Henry came in too. He was six. Simply, naturally, he gave her a kiss. "'Bye, Audrey."

And he left the room.

Aline stayed a moment longer, looking at her sister. Audrey had her eyes closed, but she noticed her presence.

"Pray for me, okay, Aline?"

"Of course. I would have done it anyway, even if you hadn't asked me to," Aline responded tenderly.

After a short while, Audrey made a great effort to lift herself up. Mummy wasn't at her side. But Mummy saw her. She helped her out of bed. Audrey walked slowly to the other side of the hallway, leaning on the wall for support. It was an immense effort for her. She went slowly, and Mummy watched her. The little ones were watching television. Audrey came closer. She said something to them, took Beatrice's little hands and caressed them. She drew near to Grégoire and caressed his head. She stayed with them a few moments and then retraced her steps and got back into the bed again. Silent tears streamed down Lillian's face. She had understood very well.

Tuesday dawned. Lillian awakened. With her head still on the pillow, she heard Audrey sing a little song from Mass. "How beautiful are your works, how great they are." Her voice sounded so exceptionally beautiful and sweet that Lillian almost didn't recognize it. It seemed like a real angel was singing, and with so much joy. She became frightened. Then Audrey said out loud:

"Ah, yes, my Lord. Thank you for having answered me so quickly."

A great fear ran through Lillian's whole body. Audrey was speaking to someone, and that "someone" was in the room. She sat up slightly, wanting to escape and flee from the room. Audrey was looking straight in front of her towards the foot of the bed. She had not realized that Mummy was awake. She didn't turn her head towards her mother. Lillian, unable to think, headed for the door and raced down the stairs in her dressing gown. Her heart was pounding. She saw Granny arranging the dining room flowers. She went towards her, but could not explain the inexplicable. A short while later, Madame Toutin, the cleaning lady, went up to leave the dresses she had ironed for Audrey in her room. She came out of the room with tears in her eyes and her face full of emotion.

"Did something happen, Madame Toutin?" asked Lillian uneasily.

"No, Madame. She just said, 'Thank you, Madame Toutin,' but her smile was so pretty and her face was all bright. I will never forget it."

It was ten in the morning.

Lord, protect me

Lillian tried to put her thoughts in order. She was agitated. They had to go to Caen. They were expecting them at the hospital for the transfusion. At the end of the morning, Audrey had fallen into a semi-coma. Lillian carried Audrey downstairs, and Granny got into the backseat of the car with Audrey at her side. They put her in with great care.

"Lord, protect me," murmured Audrey, with her eyes closed.

Lillian drove. Grandpa followed them in his car in order to bring Granny home on the return trip. During the ride, Lillian sorted through a multitude of feelings, decisions, thoughts, and memories.

"I'm bringing her to Paris. I don't want her to die away from home."

In fact, before leaving, she had asked Geoffroy, Odile's husband, to take the train to Caen so that he could then drive them back to Paris. Lillian also called her in-laws in Paris and asked them to prepare La Celle St. Cloud for their arrival. The hospital arranged for oxygen and everything that was needed to be delivered to the house within the hour. She called Marc in Bordeaux. They reached Caen and the doctors acted quickly. Transfusion and oxygen. Audrey fell into a semi-coma again. Geoffroy soon appeared at the hospital. It was a question of minutes. They put Audrey in the car again. Lillian would sit with Audrey in the back. Geoffrey drove.

I Am Entering into Life

The two-hour trip seemed never ending, but they finally arrived at the house. Mami, Dadi, Lillian, and Audrey. Silence. They kept watch and prayed. They spent the whole night like that. And Wednesday. Fatigue, tension, silence, watching, praying. Marc arrived and administered the IV and the morphine. The nurses came in twice a day. In the middle of the night, Audrey woke up for a brief moment. Lillian wet her lips with water from Lourdes.

"Thank you, Mummy."

Those were her last words.

Father Pierre arrived. He entered the room and was alone with her for a good hour. Audrey was unconscious. Father, at her side, spoke to her, prayed out loud. He also prayed in silence. The door opened. "That's it. I've entrusted everything to Audrey." He added that he had the whole Legionary seminaries of Spain and Rome praying for the girl. Some time later, he confided, full of wonder, to Lillian and Jerome: "I have seen the work of God in her."

One more night. They had already lost all sense of time. The hours went by. They needed to sleep, but it was impossible. Thursday dawned. It was August 22nd, the feast of the Queenship of Mary. Yes, it was a feast day of the Blessed Virgin. Jerome had secretly prayed, from the bottom of his heart, that Mary would give him the gift of taking his daughter on a day dedicated to her.

It would happen at three in the afternoon. Lillian and Marc were with Audrey. Marc left the room, and Mami and Dadi waited outside the room together.

It was finished.

Queen Mary had finally opened the doors of heaven for her. Now they would dress Audrey in blue, just like her queen. *We give you thanks, Lord, for so much tenderness.*

CHAPTER 6

✤

A Rain of Flowers from Heaven

"Jesus, what use are my flowers and my songs to you?… They are a perfumed rain, these songs of love from the smallest of hearts…they will make the Church Triumphant smile, and she will collect my flowers plucked out of love, and…wanting to play with her daughter, will fling them over the Church Militant so that it will win the victory."

ST. THÉRÈSE OF LISIEUX

we give you thanks for
so much tenderness

La Celle St. Cloud, August 23rd. A white truck stopped in front of the house.

"Yes?"

"An Interflora shipment from the United States."

It was an enormous bouquet of white lilies. They had been sent by a faraway relative who had heard the news.

Lillian had been hoping to find lilies for her daughter, but it had been impossible to find them at this time of year at any of the florists. Her friends Odile and Caroline had also been searching. White lilies: the sign of purity, of the Resurrection.

They were the flowers of one who had conquered a throne, the flowers of one who smiled in the arms of Mary, the Queen of Heaven. Audrey had been brought down to the chapel of the house where she lay surrounded by flowers and the Blessed Sacrament. She was wearing the crown of white silk flowers that she had worn for her first holy Communion. Her rosary was draped over her tiny fingers. A medal of Mother Mary was around her neck. It was quiet, calm, and peaceful.

August 24th, the Church of St. Joan of Arc, Versailles. In spite of the fact that many people had still not returned from their vacations, the church was full. It was also full of white flowers—and a stirring hymn: "We give you thanks for so much tenderness. You give living water through your pierced side. We bless you for so much tenderness. You give Life, you give the Spirit. You are my God, you are the one I seek, and my heart and my flesh yearn for you...."

Father Thévenin spoke. "What Jesus asks us today is that we follow the example of Audrey, accepting his will with an obedience full of love. Audrey, from the heights where she is now already living, wants it with all her strength. She will get it for us if we know how to ask for it, for the necessary graces.... Together with Audrey, let's say these words of St. Thérèse: 'I want every-thing he wants.'"

A friend who had just returned to Versailles happened to be passing by the Church. Seeing it open, he looked in. Catching sight of the small white coffin, he suddenly realized that it must be Audrey's funeral. He was struck by the atmosphere—an atmosphere where so much unspeakable pain had given way to unearthly joy and serenity. He confided to Jerome later: "I felt as if I was looking through a window into heaven."

One month later, in the Chapel of the Capuchins of Versailles, Father Thévenin celebrated a Mass for the children of the Tuesday Rosary, a Mass for Audrey's friends. They had prayed so much for her. They wanted to know, they wanted to understand why Jesus had brought her to heaven.

Dear friends of Audrey, it is above all to you, the children, that I direct these words. To begin with, we know that when one speaks to children, the adults are very happy and always learn something.

It is Audrey who reunites us today. We pray with her, who is already close to Jesus. We have done everything we could for her. Her friends have prayed a great deal for her in school and in their families.

One day, when we knew that Audrey was going to leave earth to go meet Jesus, some children said, "But I don't understand it! I had prayed so much for her that she would get well. I made so many sacrifices, and look, it has all been useless." It certainly has been useful, because God listens to all our prayers, when we make them with love. He listens to everything, especially to the prayers of children.

But God is God, and God does what he wants. We can pray with all our strength, with all our faith, with all our hope, and with all our love. If God decides that one of his children should come close to him, then he can do what he wants. And God has done what he wanted.

But be careful. Don't be mistaken; all the prayers that we said for Audrey have not been useless. First, they served to help her overcome her suffering better, so that she could offer all her sacrifices to Jesus, and that's what she did. And I am sure that all the prayers we said have helped and served other people.

God wanted to make Audrey a very beautiful soul in a hurry.

St. Thérèse of the Child Jesus, whom Audrey loved very much, wrote: "The world of souls is like the garden of Jesus. He has wanted to create great saints, who are like the lilies and the roses. But he has also created the tiny saints and these are content to be daisies or violets destined to please the eyes of God who has put them under his feet." Listen well; it is very important: "Christian perfection consists in doing His will and in being what He wants us to be."

What do we hope for from children? That they do God's will. That they do the will of their parents, of their Mummy. In a word: that they be very obedient.

God loves all the flowers. God loves all men. The smallest grow very quickly and become very beautiful in a hurry. The big ones grow less quickly and are also very beautiful, but they need more time.

Look at the great saints. You know of great saints who have founded orders, orders where there are many men and women who want to imitate them…Saint Bernard, Saint Francis. But, on the other hand, there are also all the small daisies, all the little violets, and these are Jacinta and Francisco of Fatima….

Perhaps Audrey will never be canonized. Or maybe she will be! I don't know, but what I do know is that Audrey is the little daisy or the violet. What is certain is that she wanted to live like a great Christian. She flowered. And Jesus wanted this little girl to come very close to his heart very quickly. Saint Dominic Savio, a young, fourteen-year-old saint, told Don Bosco, "I want God to make me holy, and fast." We know this sentence, but sometimes we forget what he added, "Because God could take me along the way."

On the long path of a life, there are some who die young because God grants them the grace of going more quickly than others. There are little ones who accelerate and run towards Jesus much more quickly because God attracts them to himself with great strength, and these little ones say yes to Jesus. They reach him more quickly because he has wanted it that way.

Dear little friends of Audrey, let's pray for sick children so that they will be true Christians and so that they will get well if God wants it. And if God wants them to be close to him very quickly, then let's pray that they will be holy and will go to heaven. Amen.

we don't choose the saints; they choose us

Some years ago, Lillian and the children visited a Poor Clare convent in Bordeaux. Jerome's brother, Marc, knew the sisters because he was the doctor who cared for the community. The mother Abbess confided to her visitors that she was worried about the scarcity of vocations. Not a single young woman with vocational stirrings had knocked on the door for a long time. Audrey decided to pray a lot for this intention, and at the beginning of Audrey's sickness, Lillian also called the mother Abbess to ask her for prayers for Audrey. During Audrey's sickness, this religious thanked her several times, very moved, for all that Audrey was offering for vocations. One afternoon, one of the religious saw that the photograph of Audrey that had been sitting on the altar where the community prayed had slipped onto the floor. It was August 22nd. The next week, four young women arrived at the convent asking for a retreat to discern their vocations.

A young relative of Geoffroy, Odile, and Father Jean Bernard suffered a car accident a few days before Audrey's death. He fell into a coma, and as the days went by, he didn't come out of it. They entrusted him to Audrey's intercession for a cure. Finally, the family's moment of joy arrived: he came out of the coma. It was August 22nd.

In June, Father Pierre had asked Audrey to pray for a French girl who was searching for her vocation, to pray that she would find "the right path." A few months later, she decided to become consecrated to God in the Regnum Christi movement. The date was August 22nd. Later, she discovered the "coincidence" of dates, but it was only years afterwards that she knew her vocation had been entrusted to Audrey's prayer.

A seminarian asked Audrey to pray that the Legionaries of Christ would find a school in Switzerland. A few months later, he visited the Le Châtelard Academy for the first time. The date?

August 22nd. It was only afterwards that he knew that she had died on that same day.

A young Brazilian, Victor, had leukemia the same year as Audrey. He called a Legionary priest who was thousands of miles away. He told him that he had decided to commit suicide by pulling out all the tubes that kept him alive because he didn't want to bear the pain anymore. The priest told him, "There is a girl in France who has the same thing as you. She is offering her suffering to God." He thought about her, he fought, and he got well. A few years later, this young man came to Paris to work with the Legionaries. While staying with the family in La Celle St. Cloud, he told Jerome the story without knowing who the girl was. At the end, Jerome told him, with tears in his eyes, "That girl was Audrey, and you're sitting on her bed."

Jerome gave a testimonial speech about his daughter at a seminary in Rome. At the end, one of the seminarians took him aside and told him, "Listen, I want you to know that I received a grace from God that saved my vocation, and it was through your daughter."

In 1993, an article about Audrey fell into the hands of a Legionary priest. It touched his heart. From that day, he began a spiritual friendship with her that grew until the two of them became real coworkers in the divine business. Today, for this priest, who is a spiritual guide for many consciences, Audrey is his "little Carmelite," the protector of his priestly vocation, and his great ally in his vocational apostolate.

And what happened to McLean? He was ordained a priest in the United States in 1998. During the first Mass that he celebrated he wore a very special stole: it was the tricolor scarf that Audrey had knit for him in the hospital. He is convinced that it was Audrey who saved his vocation. A few years earlier, Mick had the opportunity of greeting the Holy Father after serving as an acolyte at a Mass in the Vatican. He showed him the picture of his niece, and the Holy Father looked at it with attention, saying, "I have seen this photograph before." The Holy Father listened with interest as McLean told him about his family.

Aline had adopted, through prayer, a French seminarian who was working in Japan. Here is the letter that he wrote her after Audrey's death.

TOKYO, AUGUST 26, 1992

It has been a few days since you have received my postcard from Korea telling you about a letter on the way. I am sending you these lines en route to Japan. In October of last year, a lady invited me to one of her catechism meetings to talk to her group of children. Right before leaving my office, I got the mail and found your letter telling me about your sister's birth into heaven. On the way to the catechism teacher's house, I couldn't stop thinking and praying for you and for Audrey. I was welcomed by the joyful shouts of the children and tried to hide my pain.

The session began. We began to pray, and out of nowhere, a boy started to ask questions about death, and another started telling him all about another little boy who had died young after a sickness. I couldn't believe what I was hearing. It seemed like everything was prepared so that Audrey's story would be told. I told him what your dad had told me during our trip to Rome and everything that I remembered. I prayed to God for a sign in order to know whether or not this story was really important for this group. Two things happened:

> *One lady was very attentive and asked me, "This little Audrey—was she from Versailles?" She then explained to me that she knew her and had participated in one of the Tuesday rosary sessions.*

> *One of the boys started talking about St. Thérèse of*

Lisieux. He quoted her phrase, "I am not dying, I am entering into life." That same quotation was on the card Audrey chose in Lisieux.

I became convinced that this meeting was the work of Providence. Then I proposed to the group that we choose Audrey as our companion for the whole of that year. Everyone was in agreement. The graces have been numerous. The children have become true little missionaries. They speak easily of Jesus at school, and they have brought their little friends to the catechism group. A six-year-old boy has managed to bring his parents to Mass. His mother has asked for baptism, and she will receive the sacrament next Easter.

A few months ago, the group became associated with the Child Adorers of Montmartre.

At the end of the year, in June, the catechism teacher organized a dinner for the parents of all the children in the group. During the dinner, the lady told them all that they had lived during the year, beginning with what had happened in October when I arrived with the news of Audrey's death. While she was telling the whole story, she was asking herself, "Should I tell them all this?" The telephone rang. It was her husband from France. He was returning from Versailles, where he had just finished participating in the Tuesday Rosary, and many people had spoken to him about Audrey.

Deo Gratias...

...I don't know what you will think, but I have received all this as a gift from heaven. I pray that it will become a source of joy for you. I know that I can't begin to imagine your sadness. I ask your forgiveness if I have lacked delicacy in this letter. I want you to know that it comes from the bottom of my heart.

We are united in the heart of Jesus and Mary.

A big hug. Give my regards to your parents.

Your little brother,
Regis

My Dear,

Yes, a letter from Papa! I just wanted to let you know what Audrey has been up to lately.

When I arrived in Perpignan, I spoke about her a little, but not too much. You realize, I hope, that the company I work for now belongs to a charismatic community called "The Glorious Cross." This community's vocation is to support the parishes. They have a very beautiful liturgy, they are very close to the Pope, and their general pastor (like their general director) is an extraordinary priest, a former professor in the seminary of Saint Sulpice in Paris. Anyway, I participate in the parish life during the week, going to the 6:15 Masses and sometimes to the vigil Masses, like the one at Saint Joseph's last Tuesday.

When Christmas came, I thought about giving them a gift to thank them for all their care, especially during my operation and convalescence (Jerome had just suffered another collapsed lung.) I photocopied sixteen copies of the testimonial speech about Audrey that I gave in November in Rome. For each recipient, I added a few words and a picture of Audrey.

I was absolutely not expecting what came next. To begin with, one of the nuns had been praying to our Lord for ten years that she would find a certain prayer for vocations that she had said as a child but could no longer remember. This prayer is the "Prière à Notre Dame du Sacerdoce" which is printed on the back of the picture. You can imagine her excitement. Then the pastor told me that he had been praying to Audrey for God to send them vocations, but since last week, he decided to ask our Lord that all the vocations in the diocese come through Audrey's intercession. And this has already started. A young man came along saying he was going to Paris because it was impossible to find someone to marry in Perpignan. Last Tuesday, both the pastor and I—without consulting each other—entrusted this boy to Audrey, sensing that he had a vocation. Poor boy, he doesn't know what's in store for him. Pray for him, but be discreet, since one shouldn't light the wick before the Lord. "He needs to find the right way."

March 18 was Audrey's birthday. At 3:00 I went into the sacristy to meet briefly with the lady in charge of the offerings for the Mass. We put: "In thanksgiving for Audrey's fourteen years." I arrived at Mass around 6:00 in order to be punctual. There was an incredible commotion. All the Brothers and Sisters of the other two parishes of St. Paul of Fenouillier and of Toulouse were there. We greeted each other; we embraced each other; we congratulated each other. A real whirl! When I asked what this joyful reunion was due to, they told me that twice a year the whole community got together and one of those times was on the eve of the feast of St. Joseph.

Fourteen priests were concelebrating. The one who announces the intention of the Mass appeared in front of the altar and with open arms announced in a powerful voice (not at all his usual way of doing this) and with a tone of voice that showed to what extent he had personally committed himself: "In thanksgiving for Audrey's fourteen years." A woman parishioner near me said, "Who is Audrey?" Not knowing the answer, her neighbor shrugged his shoulders. What can I say, except that I myself and the members of the community who told me about it, saw in this coincidence that heaven had given its assent to the spiritual adoption of the community by Audrey, and vice versa. Believe me, she is in good hands. I don't know what plan of heaven is hidden behind this adoption.... It is a great mystery! The future has yet to tell us, perhaps. In any event, I believe it to be so. We are only in the beginning of our surprises, or, to be more precise, of our amazement.

Last point. Remember how Audrey loved St. Thérèse? I did a little research on her a while ago and read Story of a Soul *and two or three other things. I fell upon this prayer: "I beg you to choose a legion of small victims of Your Love." It was at the end of her life. It makes one think, doesn't it? It seems to me, as a father, that I cannot downplay the importance of what happened. At the same time, I am discovering that all this could be much greater than we imagine.*

A kiss. I think of you often.

Papa

During all this, one day Jerome shared his wonder with one of the members of the community, who responded: "Look, we are not the ones who choose the saints. It is they who choose us."

A LETTER FROM PAPA TO AUDREY

Dearest daughter,

It has been eight years since you went on ahead of us. Well, I will write it. I'm trying once again to escape it. Eight years have passed since you died. And the death of a child, here, is seen as something bad: it's called a scandal, a monstrosity. Even a mother told me one day, "You see, you believe in God and look what happened to you." Many people think God is rewarding your mother and I very little for our commitment to his Church.

It's true that our pain, and especially your mother's, is far from over. But what is this pain? It's like a storm in a barrage of sentiments that go from blind, animal pain to the purest spiritual joy. And what really hurts is the impossibility of reaching you in this sweetness of which I have a presentiment, this sweetness which is so great that no words could describe it, this sweetness which you are now fully living.

Do you remember? You were in bed, wearing your yellow flowered dress. It was one of those rare moments of your sickness when we found ourselves alone. For a long time, I was caressing your little hands, so thinned from the sickness. You were so weak that we thought you were going to die very soon. I had the sudden desire to ask your forgiveness. I started with a compliment: "You have very pretty hands." You smiled, your eyes still closed. I continued, "I haven't always been a good Papa." You smiled again and told me three words in response: "Oh, yes, Papa!" I could never find the words to express the immense sweetness contained in these three words. So very much sweetness that I realize only now, as I write them, that you too were throwing me a compliment. By these three words, my little girl…. Well, these three words will be my secret. Our secret.

What is less and less a secret (and I strongly hope that it will continue not to be one) is the specificity of your vocation—or, as the theologians call it—your "charism": the spiritual support of vocations, particularly of religious and priestly vocations. Here, with your small, strong hand, you were already directing the spiritual affairs of your family. But you seem to be adopting many new families in the process. They tell me many good things about you, and I feel very proud. In many places, they tell me that upon listening to and recounting the "Audrey stories," young people accept the urgent call of Christ.

Today, a vocation cannot be received with reason alone. There aren't enough examples. There are priests and seminarians who have chosen you as their second "Mummy." They tell me that their little Carmelite takes very good care of them. Their self-surrender is so weakened by the world that they need to support themselves by a point of reference that is very small, very sweet, and very pure.

You ask me, sometimes, to help in your undertakings. "I am not a very good Papa," but I try to do the best I can. I am at your disposal. Thanks in return for all the "Thank yous"….

I would like to give you a hug,
Your Papa

P.S. I haven't touched a cigarette for eight years… Thanks.

EPILOGUE

❦

FIFTEEN YEARS
AFTER AUDREY'S DEPARTURE
FOR HEAVEN...

Aline is a consecrated member of the
Regnum Christi Movement. Her brothers
Henry and Grégoire and her cousins Joseph,
Brigitte's son, and Paul, Marc's son,
are preparing to be priests of the
Legion of Christ.

APPENDIX

Audrey's Letters and writings

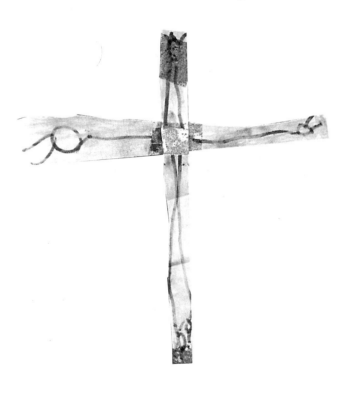

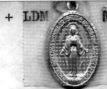

+ LDM

MISSIONARIES OF CHARITY
54A A.J.C. BOSE ROAD
CALCUTTA — 700016
Lent 1991

Dear Audrey,

This brings you God's blessing and
my prayer that you may never let
anything so frighten you or fill
you with sorrow as to make you forget that you are a child of the
Father - precious to Jesus - Temple
of His Spirit and Loved by His
Mother. Keep the joy of being lov-ed
by Jesus burning in your heart and
share this joy with all around.

When you are sad or worried, just
put yourself in the Hands of our
Lady. Ask Her to be Mother to you.
I am sending a miraculous medal for
you. Use it with the prayer:"Mary,
Mother of Jesus, make me alright".
She will take care of you.

God bless you
ee Teresa

Original letter from Mother Teresa to Audrey (received March,
1991 while Audrey was in the sterile bubble)

Previous page: one of the crosses made by Audrey, age three, for
her new home *(also featured on the cover)*

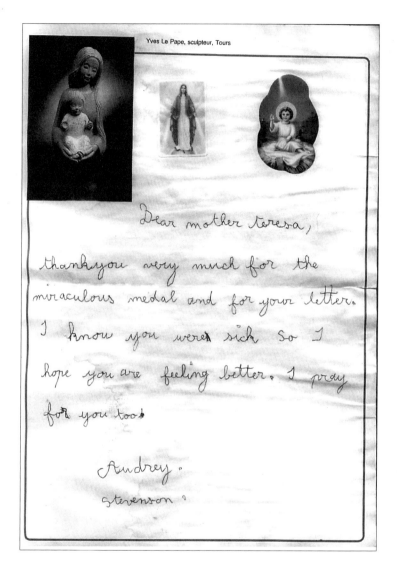

Yves Le Pape, sculpteur, Tours

Dear mother teresa,

thank you very much for the
miraculous medal and for your letter.
I know you were sick so I
hope you are feeling better. I pray
for you too.

Audrey.
Stevenson.

Original letter from Audrey to Mother Teresa

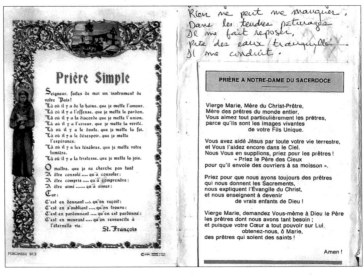

Some of Audrey's favorite prayers

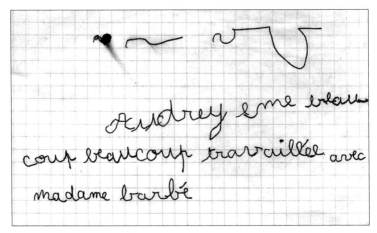

Writing exercises to recover the use of her hands after the convulsions, June 1991

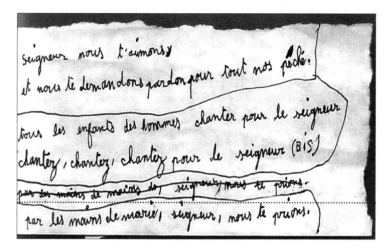

Songs composed by Audrey for the Mass on her patron saint's day, June 23, 1991

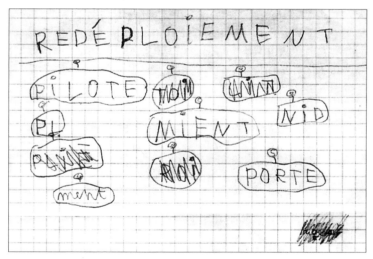

Audrey loved the challenge of doing word games, although it was more and more difficult for her to write.

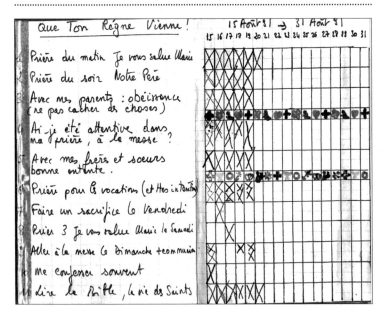

+LDM
21st July, 1993

MISSIONARIES OF CHARITY
54, A. A ᴜ C Bose Road.
Calcutta 700016 India

Dear Lillian

Thank you very much for your letter.

Yes – your daughter is much closer to you now than ever – because she is with Jesus and Jesus is in our hearts – So Audrey must be there also.
Please be assured of my prayers for your brother McLean Cummings that He become a Holy priest – only all for Jesus.

God Bless you

Mc Teresa Me

Original letter from Mother Teresa to Lillian

Que Ton Règne Vienne!

Notebook, or prayer manual, that Audrey copied from her sister Aline. Aline brought it back from summer camp, July 1991. Audrey lived it faithfully during the last twenty days of her life and made it the subject matter of her confessions.

Prière du matin

Seigneur, dans le silence de ce jour naissant, je viens Te demander la paix, la sagesse, la force.

Je veux regarder, aujourd'hui, le monde avec des yeux tout remplis d'amour. Etre patient, compréhensif, doux et sage. Voir, au-delà des apparences, tes enfants comme tu les vois Toi-Même, et ainsi ne voir que le bien en chacun.

Ferme mes oreilles à toute calomnie. Garde ma langue de toute malveillance. Que seules les pensées qui bénissent demeurent en mon esprit.

Que je sois si bienveillant et si joyeux que tous ceux qui m'approchent sentent Ta présence.

Revêts-moi de Ta beauté, Seigneur, et qu'au long de ce jour je Te révèle. Amen.

ANGE MICHEL - LYON - CCM 12

Audrey's favorite morning prayer

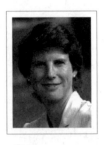

about the author

GLORIA CONDE was born in Barcelona, Spain, in 1966.
She has a bachelor's degree in journalism from the University of
Madrid and completed advanced coursework at the Francisco de
Vitoria University. She has been awarded top honors in journalism
and integral communication. She also received a bachelor's degree
in education from the Anahuac University in Mexico. For the last
fifteen years she has worked intensely as a university educator
in Italy, Switzerland, Mexico, and Spain, including working with
youth on their human and spiritual formation.

If you would like to communicate with Gloria directly,
her email address is: gconde@inteducators.org